HIPPOCRATES

PSEUDEPIGRAPHIC WRITINGS

STUDIES IN ANCIENT MEDICINE

EDITED BY

JOHN SCARBOROUGH

VOLUME 2

HIPPOCRATES

PSEUDEPIGRAPHIC WRITINGS

LETTERS—EMBASSY—SPEECH FROM THE ALTAR—DECREE

Edited and Translated with an Introduction by

Wesley D. Smith

E.J. BRILL
LEIDEN • NEW YORK • KØBENHAVN • KÖLN
1990

Library of Congress Cataloging-in-Publication Data

Pseudepigraphic writings / Hippocrates : edited and translated with an introduction by Wesley D. Smith.
p. cm. — (Studies in ancient medicine : v. 2.)
Includes bibliographical references and index.
Contents: Letters—Embassy—Speech from the altar—Decree.
ISBN 9004092900 (cloth)
1. Hippocrates—Spurious and doubtful works. 2. Medicine, Greek and Roman. I. Hippocrates. II. Smith, Wesley D., 1930- III. Series.
R126.H7A1 1990
610'.938—dc20 90-42993
CIP

ISBN 90 04 09290 0

PRINTED IN THE NETHERLANDS

for

Karen

CONTENTS

PREFACE

This is the first full scholarly text of the *Pseudepigrapha* since Littré's edition of 1861 and the first English translation ever to be published. I have utilized the texts of the papyrus manuscripts of the letters and have developed a new assessment of the epistolographic manuscript tradition and made a new collation of all important manuscripts.

These are important writings, though they have been neglected for various reasons. They are not what they pretend to be, and the mentality they express is different from a modern one. Far from answering the questions moderns have wanted answered, the *Pseudepigrapha* have appeared to confuse the subject. The ancients did not know precisely what Hippocrates wrote nor details of his life any more than we, but like us they were curious to understand by what miracle the peculiarly Greek, disciplined, rational, progressive medical profession had developed. They answered their questions not as moderns have, with theories about schools and scientific method, but with narratives, stories that embodied their best thoughts (or instincts) about human personality and historical process. Sometimes one feels that their "best thoughts" are none too good, but not seldom they seem at least as good as more impressively phrased modern insights. In any case, these pseudepigraphic writings are what survived by whatever series of accidents. They were attached to the writings collected under Hippocrates' name and developed their own history as texts.

In the many years that I have worked on these writings I have benefitted from assistance by many people and institutions. My early work on the manuscripts was supported by a grant from the National Library of Medicine. I enjoyed the hospitality and assistance of the library of the Wellcome Institute for the History of Medicine, and have received much help from the library of the University of Pennsylvania. I completed preparation of the book in London, Ontario, enjoying the hospitality of the Jason A. Hannah Institute., I received much helpful criticism from my London seminar colleagues, Paul Potter, Beate Gundert and Maury Hanson, and this is a better book for it. Phillip De Lacy read an early draft, John Graham, Ann Hanson, and John Scarborough read it all. I have used many of their corrections and suggestions. Karen Faulkner, my wife, has made critical corrections and improvements at every stage. The Humanities Computing Center at the University of Pennsylvania, and Jay Treat's instruction, made my composing the book possible. For the basic editing I used the Ibycus computer system created by David Packard, and in this I received much help from Robert Kraft and Jack Abercrombie. The book was finally composed by me on the Macintosh using Kadmos fonts, a process that gives a satisfying degree of control, and also makes me peculiarly responsible for those mistakes that remain.

ABBREVIATIONS

AJP	*American Journal of Philology.*
AM	*Athenische Mitteilungen*
BCH	*Bulletin de Correspondance Hellenique.*
BHM	*Bulletin of the History of Medicine.*
CMG	*Corpus Medicorum Graecorum.*
D-K.	H. Diels, W.Kranz, *Die fragmente der Vorsokratiker.* 10th ed., 1961.
F. Gr. Hist.	Felix Jacoby, *Fragmente der griechischen Historiker.* 1923-.
H-G	Rudolf Herzog, *Heilige Gesetze von Kos.* 1928.
HSCP	*Harvard Studies in Classical Philology.*
Kühn	Carl G. Kühn, *Claudii Galeni opera omnia,* 1821-30.
Littré	Emil Littré, *Oeuvres complètes d'Hippocrate.*,1839-1861.
NGG	*Nachrichten d. Göttingen Gesellschaft,* Phil-Hist. Klasse.
N.H.	*Naturalis Historia.*
OCD	*Oxford Classical Dictionary,* 2nd ed., ed., N.G.L. Hammond, and H.H. Scullard. Oxford: 1970
P-H	W. R. Paton and E. L. Hicks, *The Inscriptions of Cos,* 1891.
RE	*Paulys Real-Encyclopädie der classischen Altertums–wissenschaft,* Neue bearbeitung herausgeben von Georg Wissowa 1894 ff.
REA	*Revue des Études Anciennes.*
REG	*Revue des Études grecques.*
Scr. min.	*Claudii Galeni Pergameni scripta minora,* vols. 1-3, ed. J. Marquardt, I. Müller, and G. Helmreich, 1884-93.
SEG	*Supplementum Epigraphicum Graecum.*
SIG	Wm. Dittenberger, *Sylloge Inscriptionum Graecarum*³, 1920.
S-W	Susan M. Sherwin-White, *Ancient Cos,* 1978.
ZPE	*Zeitschrift für Papyrologie und Epigrafik.*

INTRODUCTION

Systematic Greek attempts to reconstruct the early history of medicine began in the Hellenistic period after the anonymous remains of early medical works had been collected under the name of Hippocrates in the Alexandrian Library, and after the profession had divided into sects, αἱρέσεις, which held distinct doctrines about methodology in medicine. Medical people who wrote histories were apt to project backward onto the early period the disputes in which they were engaged, to emphasize epistemology and methods of inference, and to try to demonstrate that they themselves were the logical end of medicine's development.[1] But medicine was of interest to other parts of the populace also, as a cultural phenomenon. It was an expression of Greek genius and Greek ethics, of Greek discipline's conquest over disorder, and it was proof of the superiority of mind and will to physical forces, and of humaneness to indifference. The subject matter of medicine is pain, difficult breathing, vomiting, urine and bowel movements, mixtures of honey and barley broth and acrid herbs, sweat, reduced diet, menstruation and lochial flows, and other undignified things unfit for literature. Yet potentially medicine's effects are as great as battles won and cities conquered. Because of its crucial effects on human lives it offered scope for mystification and for self-enrichment of the practitioners. And because the power of medicine to make a difference in most cases was ambiguous, it gave rise to popular humor about medical quibbling, obfuscation, murderousness, and greed.

Thoughtful popular literature about the nature of the profession took the form of imaginative historical dramatization such as we have in the Hippocratic Letters and speeches, which turn the profession into a personality that experiences problems and triumphs.[2] The form was congenial to the Greeks, who used it often to fill the place of literary and social commentary and historical analysis. Both the epistolary genre and the imaginative speech put into a historical setting were much used for propaganda for and against their subjects. So it is no surprise that Hippocratic pseudepigrapha were written. It is disappointing that they are virtually all that we have, that there are not even poor historical accounts to give us clues about the reality that the pseudepigrapha pretend to portray. And the very meagerness of the pseudepigrapha suggests that they are largely based on airy fancies, unlike some pseudepigraphic collections that exploit richer historical material contemporary with their subjects.[3]

---

[1] See W. D. Smith, "Notes on Ancient Medical Historiography." *BHM* 63 (1989) 73-109.

[2] In the Corpus Hippocraticum we have semi-professional rhetorical defenses of medicine from charges of intellectual emptiness and lack of success, of which the best example is π. τέχνης, *On the Science*.

[3] The Letters of Themistocles, Plato, and the Minor Socratics are rich, for example, to the extent that they exploit good material, much of which remains to us. The letters of Heraclitus are even thinner than the Hippocratic letters, presumably for lack of source material.

But these meager writings were influential. They became the standard picture of the father of medicine, whether by codifying already current stories or creating them. While probably people would not have asserted their literal accuracy, their substance was alluded to as the real story of Hippocrates. They were not in competition with other versions. Though there are minor discrepancies, the picture given by the various "lives" of Hippocrates corresponds with the pseudepigrapha. But the letters and speeches themselves are a miscellaneous lot which appears to have grown by accretion, the later additions expanding and interpreting themes from previous periods.

We read them, therefore, as literary interpretations of medicine's history and status. We relate them, as best we can, to the period of their composition and identify the influences behind them and the concerns that shaped them. The speeches and *Decree* seem to be the earliest.

Speeches, Decree

Presbeutikos

Thessalos' ambassadorial speech is a literary exercise in persuasive rhetoric. While offering variations on the formula "Unaccustomed as I am to public speaking," the speaker repeatedly draws attention to the structure and style of his speech. He points to the parts of the speech as it proceeds, and notes that his style is appropriate to his subject matter. He carefully uses the standard devices to gain the audience's respect and approval, being very clear about the good and bad, and addressing the audience's self-interest. He pays close attention to the nature of proof at each stage, including the *aitiae*, the substantial proofs of the truth of his story in the Delphian inscriptions and the Athenian gifts and crowns. He carefully marks introduction, narrative, argument and conclusion. He uses but does not overuse the rhetorical figures. The speaker plays with sounds, uses the figura etymologica frequently at the opening of sections, and throughout varies the length of his sentences. The speech has a nice formal shape which he announces at the beginning, consisting of the narration of four εὐεργεσ ίαι, the benefits or good deeds, done by the people of Cos and Hippocrates' family.

The "eldest" story, told "mythologically," as the author says, succeeds in evoking the tone of epic, or of the tales of Herodotus: a mysterious oracle brings Fawn and Gold from Cos to Delphi, and the water supply of the besieged town is discovered by the general's wallowing horse. The story reads like a tale told by Coans to fit one of their leading families, which has a Thessalian connection, into early Greek history. It is noteworthy that Pausanias (10.37.6-7) tells a different story of the Amphictyonic war, one which he presumably heard at

Delphi. According to him, Solon was summoned from Athens by the Amphictyons for help in the siege, and he poisoned the water of the besieged town, Crisa, with hellebore and thus brought down the guards with severe diarrhea. In Pausanias' story, Cleisthenes, tyrant of Sicyon, is the Amphictyonic general, while in the *Presbeutikos* the general is Eurylochus, a Thessalian of Heraclid descent. The importance of Thessaly in the *Presbeutikos* is further shown by its appearance in the later tale of the plague: Hippocrates is resident in Thessaly when he is summoned by the northern barbarians, and from Thessaly he sends his sons, son-in-law, and himself to spread the medical advice that will avoid the plague. The *Epibomios*, of course, is spoken in Thessaly.

The second tale, about Cos's self-sacrificing resistance to the Persians and Cadmus's efforts to keep the Sicilians from joining the Persian side, again reads like a corrective, Coan, version of the history of the period involved. It corrects Herodotus by describing resistance to Artemisia on the island itself.[4] It also gives a different version of the role of Cadmus from that given by Herodotus. Herodotus says that Cadmus was the agent of Gelon, sent to Delphi to treat with Xerxes if the Persians won (7.163-4), but the author of the *Presbeutikos* makes Cadmus a panhellenic patriot whose purpose was to keep Sicily on the side of the Greeks. The section on Cadmus seems rather lame in comparison to the earlier vivid description of the islanders' sufferings: Cadmus, the speaker says, did many fine things which he has not time to recall. The third tale, that of the plague, appears to be a history made up by the author of the *Presbeutikos* himself, though it could actually be a traditional story on Cos. It does not appear to be based on a historical event like the other three tales, not even a minor event highly exaggerated. While one assumes that the author knew about the Athenian plague and knew Thucydides' description of it, the substance of this story of international medical intrigue is a new departure, not based on serious historical accounts or medical texts. In later times, possibly inspired by the fantasy expressed in this work, the story developed that Hippocrates had cured, or helped to cure, the Athenian plague by purifying the air with fire.[5] But the story told here of a plague threatening from the north, presumably because it had no historical support, was virtually ignored in later times, appearing only in Pliny.[6] And the notion of mass prophylaxis against plague by dietary instructions, which the *Presbeutikos* proposes, is otherwise unexampled, though of course it is an adaptation of the standard dietetic advice that one should counteract the effects of the seasons by ordering one's regimen. The *Presbeutikos* envisions the plague as

---

[4] One would infer from Herodotus that Cos acted like the neighboring islands and contributed to Xerxes' fleet (Hdt. 7.47: All the islands sent earth and water to the Persian king; 7.99: Artemisia led Coans among others.). That Coans did join the fleet may be what the *Presbeutikos* intends to say by mentioning the "bitter bargain," too bitter to talk about. Below, page 116.

[5] Jody Rubin Pinault, "How Hippocrates cured the Plague," *J. Hist. Med. and Allied Sciences* 41 (1986) 52-75.

[6] Pliny, *Naturalis Historia* 7.37 for the plague from the north, 36.79 for the statement that Empedocles and Hippocrates used fire for certain epidemic conditions.

coming from the northwest, visiting first the Illyrians and Paeonians, who are classed as barbarian enemies of Greeks, and Greeks include Macedonians. The political alignment thus imagined may well have been inspired by the activities of Philip II of Macedon, who conquered the Paeonians and Illyrians in 359-8 B. C., and brought them under Macedonian influence.[7] The close attachment of Hippocrates' family to Thessaly which this tale employs may well be based on family rather than political history, and we need not try on the basis of it to relate the composition to a time of specially close relations between Thessaly and Cos, such as may be suggested by inscriptions from the mid-third century B. C.[8]

The final tale is Thessalos' claim that he went to Sicily with the Athenian expedition of 415-13. The imagined events are not impossible historically. This tale reads as though it is based on the narrative of Thucydides, but the author does not provide any convincing details to disarm our disbelief, while he lamely has Thessalos claim that there are great numbers of things that he could say. Thessalos says only that the task that he undertook involved misery and self-sacrifice, took three years, and was acknowledged by the gift of a golden crown from the Athenian people. Similar lack of detail keeps the dramatic date and occasion of the speech obscure, although the statement that the speech is being delivered nine years after the aborted plague sounds explicit enough. Thessalos, after returning to Cos to marry, presumably around 413, when the Sicilian expedition ended, is at the dramatic date of the speech back again in Athens pleading that the Athenians not enslave Cos, and he threatens that Cos will get the aid of Thessalians, Argives, Spartans and Macedonians. The list of potential Coan allies is based on the Heraclid descent claimed by the aristocracies, and not necessarily related to any historical moment.

Speech from the Altar, Decree

The briefer, related pieces, the *Epibomios* and the *Athenian Decree*, envision closely related situations. The *Epibomios* appears to be spoken by Hippocrates in Thessaly (no city is specified) after the Athenians have disregarded Thessalos' pleas. In language drawn from the other speech, Hippocrates is made to say that the Athenians have "put Cos in the portion of a slave" (page 109 below). The *Epibomios* is, therefore, the appeal to the Thessalians on the basis of Heraclid ties that Thessalos threatens in the *Presbeutikos*. Ludwig Edelstein argues, mistakenly, I think, that the *Epibomios* is written as though Hippocrates is a stranger in Thessaly, visiting for the first time.[9] In fact Hippocrates says that he is well known there and that his name has travelled even farther than his body. It is a courtesy to readers that he does not repeat the whole substance of the

---

[7] Account in Diodorus Siculus 16.4.
[8] Sherwin White, *Ancient Cos*, 109-110
[9] RE Suppl. 6, 1298.

Presbeutikos to illustrate his claims. Only here are the obscure figures Rhoia, Anius and Sunius mentioned in the pseudepigrapha (below, page 109), and their relevance is not obvious. Sunius, who does not otherwise figure in extant versions of the myth, and who appears in the accusative, Sunium, may be the ancestral connection the author is stretching for: the name of a part of Attica proves old ties with Asclepius' father Apollo. Such abstruseness is not out of place in this turgid, brief speech.

The *Athenian Decree* also seems to derive from the *Presbeutikos*. It fulfills the *Presbeutikos*' statement that the Athenians voted Hippocrates a golden crown and initiation into the mysteries in recognition of his services in preserving them from the plague. The *Decree* goes beyond the *Presbeutikos* in saying that Hippocrates published his writings in order to create more physicians,[10] and that he resisted the Persian King. In its list of honors, the *Decree* goes beyond the *Presbeutikos* by granting to Hippocrates perpetual dinners in the Prytaneum, and by granting Coan citizens the right to participate in the Athenian ephebeia. Absence of reference to Thessalos' service to the army in Sicily is of no significance because the dramatic date of the *Decree* precedes it.

Jody Rubin Pinault has described the formal similarity of this to actual honorary decrees, and of the gifts to Hippocrates to the ones the decrees list.[11] Her analysis of the form inclines toward judging the *Decree* as somewhat late insofar as it reflects the style of extant Athenian decrees of the third century and later. I think that we can add other evidence as well. The *Decree*'s acknowledgment of the Hippocratic Corpus might appear insignificant, but it is not. It draws our attention to the fact that the celebrations of Hippocrates and his family in the *Presbeutikos* and *Epibomios* show no consciousness of the Corpus. Whoever wrote the *Decree*, though he was probably unaware that his point of view represents such a change, has in his mind an image of Hippocrates which is shaped by a body of medical literature. Furthermore, the writer of the *Decree* has the Persian letters in his consciousness. The inclusion of the Persian king in the *Decree* implies the existence of a coherent story on that subject; that is, it refers to at least some version of letters 3-6. The *Decree*'s phrase "common enemy of the Greeks" seems to reflect the actual phrasing of letter 5. No other compelling verbal similarity argues knowledge of the letters in the form that we have them.

In sum, the *Presbeutikos* and the slightly later *Epibomios* appear to be the earliest documents of the pseudepigrapha, and to be closely tied to Coan-Thessalian relations of some kind, though perhaps only of Hippocrates' family,

---

[10] In the *Decree*, it is stated that, besides making public the precautions which his students are to publish abroad, Hippocrates published his treatises because he wanted to bring more physicians into existence: ἐξέδωκε δὲ καὶ ξυγγραφὰς ἀφθόνως τὰς περὶ τῆς ἰατρικῆς τέχνης, πολλοὺς βουλόμενος τοὺς σώζοντας ὑπάρχειν ἰατρούς. In the *Presbeutikos* it is said only that he wrote down the cure and posted it publicly in the various cities: καὶ ξυγγράφων θεραπείην ἐξετίθει περὶ τὰς πόλιας.

[11] Jody Rubin, *Biographical Fiction in the Lives of Hippocrates*, diss., University of Penna. 1983, pp. 110-111.

and to reflect the aura of Athens' past. The *Decree* is later, Athens oriented, and acknowledges the Corpus Hippocraticum and the Persian story.

The Speeches and Medical History

In trying to relate the speeches to the Hippocratic Corpus and to ancient medical history, we are trying to relate a number of unknowns to one another. The nature of medical training and medical practice at any particular time is difficult to establish, in the early period most of all; the formation of the Corpus and its relation to medical practice is a matter of much dispute and conjecture; and the history of Cos is at best shadowy. I begin with the relation of the speeches to the Hippocratic Corpus. The two speeches, the *Presbeutikos* and *Epibomios*, are listed by Erotian as part of the Hippocratic Corpus, among the works that relate to the science: *Oath*, *Law*, *On the Art*, *On Ancient Medicine*; but he distinguishes the speeches from the rest with the remark that they show Hippocrates more as a patriot (φιλόπατρις) than as a physician. Erotian's work is based on a series of collections of Glossae, dictionaries of rare and interesting words in the Corpus, that had begun in Alexandria where the Hippocratic collection likely came into being, and so Erotian's testimony probably testifies to the existence of these two speeches in Alexandria, possibly in the last quarter of the third century B.C.[12] It also indicates that the speeches were transmitted with the medical works, and conversely, because the letters are not mentioned in Erotian's discussion, we may suspect that, whatever their date of composition, the letters were added to the collection of medical works at a time later than the two speeches. My reasoning here perhaps requires defense, since Herzog's assertion that the *Presbeutikos*, *Epibomios*, and *Decree* must have appeared in an Alexandrian catalogue has rightly been dismissed as mistaken.[13] Despite the meagerness of our knowledge of the early glossographies, we do know from Erotian's discussion of his predecessors that the tradition was continuous beginning from Bacchius, and it looks as though Erotian had direct access to Bacchius' *Glossae* in the composition of his own work. Erotian rejects *Prorrhetic 2* as spurious, for reasons that he does not state, but mentions no other spurious works. It is likely that his rejection of *Prorrhetic 2* is based on the work's ambiguous status in the tradition. While he says of the *Presbeutikos* and

[12] For the dating of the various glossographers see Max Wellmann, *Hippokratesglossare*, *Quellen und Studien zur Geschichte der Naturwissenschaften und der Medizin* 2 (1931). We have no direct evidence for Bacchius' glosses on the *Presbeutikos* and *Epibomios*, but it is only fortuitous when Erotian specifically quotes Bacchius' gloss of any word along with subsequent glossographers' criticisms of Bacchius.

[13] Edelstein, RE Sup. 6, 1305, 1-10. There is no evidence for an Alexandrian catalogue listing medical works.

Epibomios that they are not properly medical works, he indicates no suspicion of them. One may suspect that if he had grounds for rejecting them, such as their absence from Bacchius' *Glossae*, he would have done so.[14]

It does not seem to me possible to find a precise moment in time at which to place the composition of the *Presbeutikos* according to the view of Greece it shows. As I suggested above, its version of Greek political alignment, the status of Macedonians, Paeonians and Illyrians, suggests a time after the mid-fourth century. One cannot even exclude, probably, the periods when Athens was relatively helpless and not imperial, because the memory of Athens' greatness in Hippocrates' time, and the memory of the moral problems associated with her empires were adequately preserved in literature. The *Presbeutikos* is not propaganda aimed at influencing great states, but is rather an attempt by a family from a minor state to place itself in history. It dramatizes Cos as an innocent victim with a history of political neutrality, reminiscent of Melos in Thucydides (5.84-114). It is credible, then, that the two speeches were composed between 350 and 250 B.C.

The two speeches arrived in Alexandria and became part of the Corpus Hippocraticum with the anonymous medical works that were assembled under Hippocrates' name. It remains a mystery how and over what period of time the Corpus itself, so heterogeneous and of diverse qualities and points of view, came into being. The nearest thing to an explanation that we have is an account written at the library in Alexandria: Zeuxis, an early second century B.C.[15] commentator on works of the Corpus said that medical works on ships coming into Alexandria were seized and copied and stacked in a room or rooms for later incorporation into the Library.

> And, they say, the Ptolemy who was then king of Egypt became so greedy for books that he ordered that the books of everyone who arrived by ship be brought to him. After he had them copied on new paper he gave the copies to the owners of the books that had been brought to him on the debarkation, and deposited the confiscated books in the library with the inscription "Of those from the ships."

Shortly later he says,

---

[14] For further discussion see W. D. Smith, *The Hippocratic Tradition*, 199-204. When I wrote that, I was uncertain whether the *Presbeutikos* and *Epibomios* were in the original collection in Alexandria. I am now convinced that they must have been.

[15] There has been some discussion of Zeuxis' date. Karl Deichgräber, *Die griechische Empirikerschule*, 2nd. ed. (Berlin: 1965) 263, placed him in the first century, but that has been corrected by Fridolf Kudlien, RE II.19 (1972), cols. 386-7, and Jutta Kollesch, *Der Kleine Pauly* 5 (1975) 1527.

> The king's agents inscribed the names of all the travelers on the books that were put in storage, because they did not take the books straight to the library, but stored them in houses in heaps.[16]

The medical works collected into the Corpus are stubbornly anonymous, giving few hints about the histories of the authors or the circumstances of composition.[17] The two speeches, it appears, provided the only biography and history transmitted with the collection. It is a compelling possibility that these tales of Hippocrates, when added to the anonymous medical works, had the effect of identifying the whole as the writings of Hippocrates. The Hippocratic Corpus was first edited in the first century A.D. by Dioscurides and Capiton, who were the first to do extensive *Echtheitskritik* on the collection. It was obvious to them that the works were not all by one author, but they had no information about their sources. As so often in Greek historical and literary scholarship, the reasonable solution, in the absence of evidence, was put forth as the true one. Their imaginative solution was to use the story about Hippocrates' family and Coan medical succession to conjecture authors for the works in the collection which they could not credit to Hippocrates. They conjectured that the surgical works were early, before the time of the Great Hippocrates, that the "best and most useful" works were by Hippocrates, and that Hippocrates' sons acted as his literary executors after his death and interpolated some passages. Further, works were conjecturally attributed to the sons, son-in-law, and grandsons, who would naturally bear the name Hippocrates.[18] Though they celebrate Cos and Hippocrates' family, the two speeches themselves are silent about medical literature, a fact that makes good sense if they were composed before the Hippocratic Corpus existed. The fact that they were in the Corpus accounts for the authority their information exerted in interpretation of the Corpus.

---

[16] φιλότιμον δὲ περὶ βιβλία τὸν ⟨τό⟩τε βασιλέα τῆς Αἰγύπτου Πτολεμαῖον οὕτω γενέσθαι φασίν, ὡς καὶ τῶν καταπλεόντων ἁπάντων τὰ βιβλία κελεῦσαι πρὸς αὐτὸν κομίζεσθαι καὶ ταῦτ' εἰς καινοὺς χάρτας γράψαντα διδόναι μὲν τὰ γραφέντα τοῖς δεσπόταις, ὧν καταπλευσάντων ἐκομίσθησαν αἱ βίβλοι πρὸς αὐτὸν, εἰς δὲ τὰς βιβλιοθήκας ἀποτίθεσθαι τὰ κομισθέντα, καὶ εἶναι τὴν ἐπιγραφὴν αὐτοῖς "Τῶν ἐκ πλοίων".... καὶ τῶν ἄλλων ἁπάντων τῶν καταπλεόντων ἅμα βιβλίοις ἐπέγραφον οἱ τοῦ βασιλέως ὑπηρέται τὸ ὄνομα τοῖς ἀποτιθεμένοις εἰς τὰς ἀποθήκας. οὐ γὰρ εὐθέως ⟨εἰώθεσαν⟩ εἰς τὰς βιβλιοθήκας αὐτὰ φέρειν, ἀλλὰ πρότερον ἐν οἴκοις τισὶ κατατίθεσθαι σωρηδόν. Galen, *Comm. in Hipp. Epid. III*, ed. Ernst Wenkebach, CMG V 10, 2.1, p. 79 (Kühn 17A 606-7). In this passage Zeuxis discusses a copy of *Epidemics 3* that was apparently brought to Alexandria by Mnemon of Sidon.

[17] Sometimes author's concerns show through: the author of *Generation / Nature of the Child* is careful to cross-reference his other writings by title (cf. Iain Lonie, *The Hippocratic Treatises 'On Generation', 'On the Nature of the Child', 'Diseases IV'* [Ars Medica II.7, Berlin: 1981] 51-52. The author of *Fractures / Joints* speaks of the sins of his colleagues (see, e.g., Littré 4.182-184), and the author of *Epid.* 5 recounts his own mistakes (see. 5.27, Littré 5.226).

[18] See *The Hippocratic Tradition* pp. 235-239.

It remains puzzling how it happened that it was not known precisely what the Great Hippocrates had done and written, but yet his fame was augmented by stories like those in the pseudepigrapha. It does seem likely that there are in the Corpus writings by Hippocrates, and other writings from Cos besides the two speeches. It seems likely that the works that became the Hippocratic Corpus did not arrive in Alexandria as Hippocratic writings, but became so there: nor did the works arrive with their various authors known, but have that authorship stolen in the Library. It is apparent, therefore, that the works arrived piecemeal, as in Zeuxis' description, and that the Corpus does not represent the library of a Coan school, at least not a library that was in order and transferred in an orderly fashion like the texts of the tragedies from Athens. The works of the Corpus are therefore simply anonymous pre-Alexandrian medical works, and we can draw no direct inferences from them about Cos in Hippocrates' lifetime. If the Corpus cannot be invoked as the evidence for a flourishing scientific medical school on Cos in the Classical Period, we must inquire what is behind the stories of Hippocrates and his invention of medical science, and try to separate those descriptions of Hippocrates which are simply descriptions of the Corpus Hippocraticum from other, conceivably more substantial, evidence. One even has to ask, was there a Coan school?

The existence in a later period of some sort of formal state sponsorship of physicians on Cos is indicated by epigraphic dedications from states that had requested physicians from Cos and who expressed gratitude for their services in decrees, of which copies were erected on stones in the Coan Asclepieion. The earliest of them is from the third century.[19] For the preceding period we have no such evidence, and nothing of the kind is suggested by the *Presbeutikos* and *Epibomios*. The traditional picture of the Coan medical school has largely been a projection backward of the situation in the second century B.C. and after. Susan Sherwin White has made a very useful collection of the material from Cos, including a list of personal names from inscriptions and elsewhere, and I shall freely refer to her work.[20] However, she gives the outdated traditional description of the old Coan school of Asclepiadae, an exclusive group defined by blood ties, and she sprinkles her discussion with suggestive phrases: there was a "medical centre" on Cos, the Cnidian "local medical school had largely ceased to function by the end of the fourth century" (which is when our clear evidence begins), and so on.[21] But the evidence that she herself gives seems to point in a different direction: all the epigraphic documents we have from Cos indicate a broad and open medical profession, while control of the profession by the Asclepiadae is nowhere evidenced. No physician is ever called an Asclepiad in an inscription.

---

[19] A physician Hermias, who was honored by Cnossos and Gortyn, and the same man, perhaps, also by Halicarnassus. Susan M. Sherwin White, *Ancient Cos* (Göttingen: 1978) 267-8, and Louis Cohn-Haft, *The Public Physicians of Ancient Greece* (Northampton, Mass.: 1956) 66-7.

[20] Susan Sherwin White, prev. note. Henceforth, S-W.

[21] S-W 256-274. In her reconstruction of the early Coan school she generally follows P. M. Fraser, *Ptolemaic Alexandria*, vol. 1, Oxford: 1972, 343-4.

The doctors of Cos are named as composite groups in two inscriptions, one of which delineates their privileges at a sacrifice and the other of which concerns ritual purifications in the cult of Demeter.[22] Physicians were sent officially by the Coan ecclesia to states that requested them. Decrees honoring such physicians were erected on Cos (at the Asclepieion, which is why we have so many), thanking the physicians for dedicated service and for saving lives. Sherwin White gives profiles of ten physicians of the third and second centuries who can be identified from the inscriptional evidence.[23] One, at least, may be from Hippocrates' family. A Hippocrates, son of Thessalos, who was a physician, was honored by a foreign state (name not preserved) for his good will and medical service, around 200 B.C.[24] In addition, a wealthy man named Hippocrates lent money to the state of Calymnus in the mid-fourth century, and a Hippocrates, son of Thessalos, contributed to a wartime collection of money around 200 B.C.[25]

The way Sherwin White puts it (262-3) is, "The koinon of Coan Asclepiadai no longer provided the institutional framework of the Coan physicians." And among the reasons she considers, "The introduction in Cos of the idea of payment for teaching, which implied a widening of the traditionally family basis of the medical profession, contributed in the end to undermine the continuance and viability of a professional koinon the membership of which depended exclusively upon descent." But we should recognize that there is no evidence for that ancient status of the koinon of Asclepiads, from inscriptions or from the *Presbeutikos*, our oldest literary source that touches on the subject. The notion of a koinon which ran a school and controlled access to the profession was never held by anyone in antiquity, but is a modern inference based on several things from antiquity, of which the following seem to me to have contributed most:

1. Lack of any early medical literature other than that attributed to Hippocrates. This produced such statements as that Hippocrates invented the science, or brought it to perfection from an inchoate form,[26] that he was the first to write, that he separated medicine from philosophy,[27] etc.
2. The description of Hippocrates' family in the *Presbeutikos*, and the prominence of the Asclepiadae.
3. The promises made by the oathtaker in the Hippocratic *Oath*: To hold the teacher equal to his own parents and his children as brothers; to teach his own sons, the teacher's sons, and pupils who have signed the covenant, but no one else.[28]

---

[22] H-G 1 (P-H37) and H-G 8, both in S-W p. 263.
[23] S-W 266-270.
[24] Text in Jost Benedum, "Griechische Artzinschriften," ZPE 25 (1977) 272-274.
[25] S-W p. 269.
[26] See the Hippocratic Letter 2, and the Pseudo-Galenic *Introductio*, Kühn 14.674-676.
[27] E.g., Celsus, *De medicina* Proeme 8
[28] Edelstein's analysis of the oath as a document from a small religious sect, Pythagorean influenced, has not gained universal acceptance, but no one now would attribute the oath to

4. Galen's inferences from the above, and from his own peculiar version of medical history, which claimed that Hippocrates knew everything, including anatomy, at the very beginning. In his *Anatomical Procedures* at the opening of Book 2, he conjectures why no Anatomies were written before Diocles in the fourth century. His answer is that while medical education was in the family people practiced dissection under parental instruction from childhood. But when people outside the family were instructed in medicine as adults, things changed, education became poorer. "Hence the Art, being no longer exclusive to the Asclepiad family, was ever degenerating from one generation to the next. Thus, too, arose a demand for memoranda to preserve knowledge."[29] Galen's imaginary version is based on false premises about Hippocrates' anatomical knowledge, and is his own construct. But it has been taken as primary evidence about the Coan school. People cite it, and they do not cite anything else, because there is nothing.
5. Plato, in the *Protagoras* (311-312b), says that Hippocrates teaches for money. Moderns have embellished that, and say that he introduced the practice, was the first to do so. Sherwin White says that Hippocrates' acceptance of money was a precedent, somehow inferring it from Plato, though Plato says nothing of the sort.[30]

The works of the Corpus itself refute the notion of a restricted gentilitial practice, because the authors refer to other physicians whose theories and practice they disapprove, and give the impression of a broad and open profession, and it is clear that, since there were no legal restrictions on the practice of medicine, even a family sworn to secrecy could not have kept medical practice to itself. It is worth noticing that there was another interpretation of the early medical craft which had a vogue in antiquity and early modern times, also based on the word Asclepiad: Asclepiad was interpreted as priest of Asclepius, and it was imagined that the Asclepiads practiced medicine at the temples, and that scientific medicine developed out of priestly medicine practiced in the temples. A story based on these ideas said that Hippocrates got his methods of treatment from copying the dedications in the temple of Asclepius which told of the god's procedures.[31] What these interpretations really tell us is that the situation in the craft of medicine in the period before the assembly of the Hippocratic Corpus was a mystery because there were no writings about it, and the Corpus was of little help in creating reliable history.

Hippocrates or say that it represents the generality of the medical profession, on Cos or elsewhere. Ludwig Edelstein, *The Hippocratic Oath*, BHM Suppl. 1 (1943), rep. in *Ancient Medicine*, , ed. by O. Temkin and C.. L. Temkin, Baltimore: 1967, 3-63. Cf., e.g., Fridolf Kudlien, "Medical Ethics and Popular Ethics," *Clio Medica* 5 (1970) 107-111.

[29] *Anat. Admin.*, Kühn 2.280-281. Trans. Charles Singer, *Galen on Anatomical Procedures*, London: 1956, p. 31.

[30] S-W. p. 261.

[31] Pliny, *N. H.* 29.2, Strabo, 657 = XIV.19.

It will be useful to look at historical information we have for comparison with the *Presbeutikos* and *Epibomios*. No contemporary writings from Cos are preserved, and our knowledge of Coan history is sketchy. In the absence of local Coan histories, we depend on inscriptions and on occasional mentions in ancient historical sources.[32] In the latter part of the fifth century, Cos was a part of the Athenian Empire, paying money into the empire's treasury at Athens and subject to the vicissitudes of the war between Athens and Sparta and also to the machinations of the Persian king and his satrap who was in charge of Caria, the area of modern Turkey opposite Cos. In the years approaching the dramatic date of the *Presbeutikos* and *Epibomios*, Cos suffered a number of upheavals. In 412, Meropid Cos, a city probably in the northeastern part of the island, which had recently been devastated by an earthquake that Thucydides (8.41.2) calls "the largest in our memory," was sacked by the Spartan general Astyochus. In 411, Alcibiades, on behalf of the Athenians, built fortifications there and put an Athenian governor in place. We lack details of Cos's position in the following years, which include the date at which the *Presbeutikos* is set, but after the Athenian defeat in 405, Cos apparently became allied with Sparta, and in 394 was detached from Sparta by the fleet of the Athenian Conon and the Persian satrap Pharnabazus. Cos must have made some accommodations with the new Athenian Confederacy in the Aegean in 377, though it does not appear in the list of the confederacy's members. In 366, possibly following civil strife on Cos, the whole island was organized into a single governmental unit with its seat on the northeast coast in the city of Cos. The change probably involved a considerable removal of population and activity to the new city from Astypalaea at the other end of the island, the place that we might imagine was where Hippocrates was born, but from which there are few material remains.[33] In 357 Cos joined the ruler of Caria, Mausolus, along with Rhodes, Chios and Byzantium, in war against Athens. After Mausolus' death his wife Artemisia assumed his position. During Alexander's conquests Cos was liberated from Carian control by Macedonian forces in 332, and after the division of Alexander's empire was associated with the Ptolemies until after 200, from which time it was tied to Rome. Beginning about 300, the Asclepieion outside the city of Cos was made an important shrine, and an international festival, to be celebrated each five years, was established there in 242. One would assume that the Asclepiad clan was instrumental in caring for it and promoting it. The information is not full, but at least we can get a sense of a continuity.

---

[32] Intriguing evidence has come to light about a local Coan Epic, *Meropis*, of the late sixth century. It appears to have narrated Heracles' visit to Cos and his battle with the Meropids. See Ludwig Koenen and Reinhold Merkelbach, "Apollodoros (περὶ θεῶν), Epicharm und die Meropis," in *Collectanea Papyrologica*, ed. Ann Ellis Hanson, part 1 (Bonn: 1976) 1-26.

[33] G. E. Bean and I. M. Cook, "A Walking Tour," *Annual of the British School at Athens* 52 (1957) 119-127.

Hippocrates as known in Athens, Alexandria, Rome		*Events in Cos*
	400	
		Cos allied with Athens, 430-405, and 380-330, with considerable gaps.
Hippocrates' method is described by Plato (*Phaedrus*).		
Aristotle speaks of Hippocrates the great, and elsewhere mentions a Coan oligarchic revolution (*Politics 1304 b, 1326a*)		366 Synoecism of the island, establishment of Cos city.
346 Demosthenes says Cos under Carian control (5.25)		353 Artemisia, (widow of Mausolus) rules Cos from Caria. Her head on Coan coins (?)[34]
Menon's medical doxography features Hippocrates.		332 Cos taken by generals of Alexander the Great. Critodemus, an Asclepiad, Alexander's physician (Arrian, *Anab.* 6.11.1)
310 Hippocrates, son of Draco, physician to Roxane, killed along with her.		
		315-190 Cos in close relations with Ptolemaic Egypt
	300	
Praxagoras of Cos, teacher of Herophilus, an Asclepiad, fl. ca. 300.		ca. 300 Monument at Delphi put up by the koinon of Asclepiadae of Cos and Cnidos.
300-200, The Alexandrian Library was established and the Hippocratic Collection made.		300-250 Building of the Asclepieion on Cos.
		ca. 250 Coans establish relations with the Thessalian koinon.[35]
250-200, Xenocritus of Cos, first glossographer of the Hippocratic Corpus, followed by the *Glossae* of Bacchios		242 Asclepieia festival initiated as an international event.
	200	
		200 Hippocrates, son of Thessalos, praised on a Coan monument.

[34] See the account of this dispute, S-W 76 n. 241.

[35] Inscription published by M. Segre, *Riv. Philol.* N.S. 12 (1934) 169-193. The occasion of the decree seems to be that the Coans have established an arrangement for the importation of grain from Thessaly, and are grateful for Thessalian concessions.

		After 200 Cos becomes dependent on Rome, but is a *civitas libera*. Asclepius on Coan coins.
	100	
Apollonius admires "most divine Hippocrates." Cato deprecates Hippocrates' attitude to barbarians.		Cos's status of *civitas libera* abolished under Caesar Augustus
	I AD	
Erotian mentions the *Presbeutikos* and *Epibomios*. Scribonius Largus mentions the Hippocratic *Oath*.		53 A.D. Emperor Claudius grants immunity from taxation (Tacitus, *Ann.* 12.61). Xenophon of Cos, an Asclepiad, is Claudius' personal physician, and virtual ruler in Cos. Hippocrates on Coan coins.
	100	
	200	
ca. 200, First scholarly edition of the Hippocratic Corpus		

I return now to discussion of the status of the Asclepiads in relation to the medical profession. Important to discussion of the subject has been a monument that was set up at Delphi in the fourth century B.C by the koinon of the Asclepiads of Cos and Cnidos, on which is inscribed a copy of a decree passed by members of the koinon which defines its members as Asclepius' descendants in the male line and speaks of their privileges at Delphi. Presented first by Jean Bousquet, it was republished by Franciszek Sokolowski in something like the following form.[36]

Ἔδοξε Ἀσκλαπιαδᾶ-	The koinon of the
ν τῶι κοινῶι Κώιων	Coan and Cnidian
καὶ Κνιδίων· τὸν ἀφ-	Asclepiads decrees:
ικνεύμενον Ἀσκλα-	any Asclepiad who
πιάδαν ἐς Δελφούς,	comes to Delphi, if
αἴ κα χρήζηι τῶι μα-	he wishes to consult
ντείωι χρῆσθαι ἢ θ-	the oracle or sacrifice,

[36]Jean Bousquet, "Inscriptions de Delphes," *BCH* 80 (1956) 579-593. Franciszek Sokolowski, *Lois sacrées des cites grecques*, Supplement (Paris: 1962) No. 42. It was published also in SEG 16.326, where the conjectural restorations are different in some particulars. See also Heinrich Pomtow, "Delphische Neufunde, III. Hippokrates und die Asklepiaden in Delphi," *Klio* 15 (1918) 303-338.

ύεν, ὀμόσαντα χρῆσ- θαι ἔμεν 'Ασκλαπ[ιά]- δας κατὰ ἀνδρο[γέν]- ειαν...Ω\ - - - - ΟΙ- - - - Γ- - - -	must do so only after swearing that he is an Asclepiad by the male line.......
[lacuna]	[Stone badly worn and broken in this area]
ὃς δ[έ κα ποιῆι παρὰ] ταῦτα, μ[ὴ .μεν αὐτῶ]- ι εἴσοδον ἐ[ς τὸ μαν]- τεῖον καθάπε[ρ 'Ασκ(λ)]- απιάδαις, μηδὲ, [αἴ τ]- ι ἄλλο γέρας δίδο[τ]- [α]ι 'Ασκλαπιάδα(ι)ς πα- [ρ]ὰ Δελφῶν, μὴ δίδοσ- [θ]αι, αἴ κα μὴ ποιῆι κ- [ατ]ὰ τὰ γεγραμ(μ)ένα.	and he who acts contrary to these things should not have access to the sanc- tuary in the manner of the Asclepiads, and, if any other privilege is accorded Asclepiads by the Delphians, he should not be given it if he does not act according to what has been written.

The stone is broken in the middle and the upper and lower pieces do not fit together, and it is again broken at the bottom, though its top is intact. One cannot tell how much text is missing, but, since it is stoichedon, the number of missing letters in the damaged lines is clear. The stone says, pretty clearly, that the Asclepiads' koinon had privileges at Delphi, and that they were closely guarded. Perhaps the middle of the stone, which was worn away when it was used as a paving block, told what the privileges accorded to the Asclepiads were, and scholars have discussed the possibilities of *promanteia* and *prothysia*, the right to go to the head of the line, and to be exempt from preliminary taxes, etc. Other decrees relating to koinons give them security from taxes or from being drafted for military service in foreign states.[37] The koinons were associations of various kinds, groups of worshippers, guilds of craftsmen, federations of states, groups of magistrates.[38] Koinons of Asclepiasts, worshippers of Asclepius, functioned and left monuments in Athens, Colyphon, and elsewhere. Louis Robert properly argued that there are no grounds for connecting Asclepiasts with the medical profession.[39] Similar conclusions apply to the koinon of Asclepiads that erected this stone. The stone shows that the Asiatic koinon of Asclepiads

---

[37] A. W. Pickard-Cambridge, *The Dramatic Festivals of Athens* (Oxford: 1953) 315-319 presents such decrees relating to the koinon of artists of Dionysus.

[38] Coan inscriptions include a decree by a guild of caterers, P-H 131, a guild of worshipers of Zeus Hyetios, P-H 382, and the mention of the koinon of Asia which held games at Pergamum, P-H 104.6.

[39] Louis Robert, two articles entitled "Décret des Asclépiastes de Kolophon": *REA* 28 (1926) 7-9, and *Revue de Philologie* Ser. 3., 8 (1934) 272-4.

had a special relationship with the Delphian sanctuary, and it is likely that reciprocal privileges were extended at Asclepiad centers in Cos and Cnidos, the best known of which is the Asclepieion on Cos. It seems obvious that the Asclepiads would have been involved in setting up and maintaining the Asclepieion in Cos, as well as in promoting the pentaëteric international festival and games that were held at the Asclepieion, and which were fully established in the mid-third century. It was always the policy of Delphi to maintain cordial relations with noble families. The Asclepiads of Rhodes claimed to have been the early kings of Rhodes,[40] while the *Presbeutikos* makes the same claim for the Asclepiads of Cos. It appears, then, that this document is only indirectly related to the history of medicine, but it does shed light on the *Presbeutikos* because it is a record of the Asclepiads whom the *Presbeutikos* celebrates. Bousquet was inclined to think that the stone validated the *Presbeutikos* as a historical document by testifying to the reality of the renewal of ancient relations between Cos and Delphi in Hippocrates' time, perhaps by Hippocrates himself.[41] But that is not what it shows: rather than showing that the myths of the *Presbeutikos* are all true, the stone verifies only that the myths were told against a background of a noble Asclepiad clan.

What of these Asclepiads and the medical profession? At least from the time of Hippocrates the name Asclepiad is associated with the medical profession. Theognis and Euripides use Asclepiadae to mean medical men. They do not mean Asclepius' sons, or members of the aristocratic family in Ionia, they mean scientific medical men, as they conceived them.[42] Plato uses "Asclepiads" freely to refer to physicians.[43] Theopompus, in an aside in his history, said that the physicians of Cos and Cnidos were Asclepiads, descendants of Podaleirios, who settled in Syrnos after the Trojan war.[44] Plato, referring to Hippocrates, says, "he of the Asclepiads" to make clear which Hippocrates he means. Specifications of specific individuals as Asclepiads, however, come quite late in time, and are rare. Arrian describes Critobulus, physician to Alexander of Macedon, as "a Coan physician, of the Asclepiad family," when he reports that his sources disagree as to whether Critobulus removed an arrow from Alexander, or whether it was done by Perdiccas, Alexander's bodyguard.[45] Galen, in different places, specifies that Ctesias and Praxagoras were Asclepiads.[46] However, no physician is ever called an Asclepiad in inscriptions, whether tombstones or honorary inscriptions, nor in the literary epitaphs in the Greek Anthology, so far as I know, with one

---

[40] Aelius Aristides, 'Ροδίοις περὶ ὁμονοίας, 568.30-32 (ed. Dindorf).

[41] See the Presbeutikos p. 114, lines 31-35.

[42] Euripides, *Alcestis*, 968-70, Theognis 431-3.

[43] E.g., *Republic* III, 405-406. Plato contrasts the rough and ready medicine of the original sons of Asclepius with the degraded medicine of the Asclepiads of his own day.

[44] F. Gr. Hist. 115 F103 (14), from Photius' summary of Theopompus. "He says that the physicians of Cos and Cnidos are Asclepiads, and the earliest of them came from Syrnos, descendants of Podaleirius."

[45] ἰατρὸν Κῷον, τὸ γένος τῶν Ασκληπιάδῶν, *Anabasis* 6.11.1

[46] 10.28 Kühn, *Meth. med.*, and 18a.731 Kühn, the commentary on *Joints*.

exception that I have found, which in effect shows what could have been done, and what we are missing. That is an epitaph from Phrygia of the 2nd century A.D. (i.e., the period of Galen and Arrian), in which the dead man's family has given him the title of Asclepiad, apparently because of his father's status as physician, but possibly from the claim of family descent. The family adds the claim that he has gone off to Asclepius' medical school in the sky (or the underworld).[47]

> Μιλητουπούλιος κεῖμαι | νέκυς,'Αττικὸν αἷμα, |
> ὠκυμόρου τύχης πείσ|ματα λυσάμενος, |
> ἰητροῦ πατρὸς ὢν 'Ασκλη|πιάδης, ἐλεεινά |
> μητρὶ κασιγνήτῳ τε ἄλ[γ]|εα λειπόμενος· |
> ἀλλ''οἱ μὲν κλαίουσιν, ἐγὼ | δ' ἐνὶ παισὶ κάθημαι |
> [ἀ]θανάτων Φοίβου παι[δὶ] | διδασκόμενος.

> I lie dead here, a Miletopolitan citizen, of Athenian blood, freed from the bonds of Chance, which brings swift doom. I was an Asclepiad, my father was a physician. I leave for my mother and brother painful grief, but I, myself, sit among the children of the gods, getting instruction from Apollo's son.

Thus, Asclepiad could be used generically for physician, and some physicians, as well as non-physicians, also claimed to belong to Asclepius' family. But there are no signs of exclusivity in the medical profession based on family status. We have fourth and third century inscriptions from Cos relating to groups of physicians, and they simply speak of the doctors, *toi iatroi*.[48] Sherwin White, puzzled by the phenomenon, follows P. M. Fraser in deciding that the early guild of the Asclepiads must have lapsed.[49] We should correct that long-standing but baseless claim, and say instead that people were ready to make their name a poetic byword for physician because of Asclepius himself, but the Asclepiadae were not the whole of the medical profession, even on Cos, nor were they all physicians. The *Presbeutikos* helped the family of Hippocrates to put an impress on people's thoughts about medical history. One did not have to believe its assertions in detail in order to believe that Hippocrates and the Asclepiads were quite impressive.

To summarize, then, the *Presbeutikos* and *Epibomios* are a species of propaganda for the Asclepiads and Cos. Their introduction into the Hippocratic Corpus, in the absence of good biographical and historical information about

---

[47] Published by Werner Peek, Griechische Vers-inschriften I (Berlin: 1955)718. Earlier, A. Bessett, BCH 25 (1901) 327f.,6; W. Peek, AM 66 (1941) 81f., 24; J. and L. Robert, REG 55 (1942) 356, 146.

[48] H-G1 (P-H 37) and H-G9. See S-W p. 263.

[49] S-W 262-3.

early medicine, had much to do with the characterization of early medicine that became common in antiquity and has received new wrinkles in modern times.

The Persian Letters

In letter 3, the king of Persia, Artaxerxes, wants Hippocrates to come to his court, because good men are hard to find. The phrasing of letter 3, "It is not easy to find men δυνάμενοί τι κατὰ συμβουλήν" probably has a general sense, "men worth consulting." The king's invitation to Hippocrates is an offer to set him up as a rich Persian noble in exchange for his company, and Hippocrates' reply speaks to that invitation, putting himself and his science above concern for riches, but he adds the statement that he should not cure Persians from disease because they are enemies of Greeks. The king's response in letter 8 is a furious threat, and the Coans, who take seriously the threat that they will be wiped from the earth, give a brave and pious answer. Letters 1 and 2 stand somewhat apart. They are more expansive in style and introduce other dimensions to the exchange. In letter 1, the Persian king is desperate. He writes to Paitos, possibly Petos,[50] to whom he has given many gifts, and asks for a natural or scientific remedy for a plague, which he characterizes as a beast besmirching flocks and, probably a reflection of the *Iliad*, as dart after dart. He wants to scourge the plague: are we to recall Xerxes having the Hellespont whipped (Hdt. 7.35)? The flowery response of Paetus/Petus in letter 2 gives Hippocrates a heroic genealogy from the gods but also shows an interest in the history of the *techne* of medicine and creates some new terminology for it: Hippocrates moved medicine from minor and individual activities to large and scientific-technical ones: ἐκ μικρῶν καὶ ἰδιωτικῶν εἰς μεγάλα καὶ τεχνικὰ προήγαγε τὴν ἰητρικήν. Natural diseases are resolved by nature, science must cure epidemic ones. The method of the science in curing plague is to judge the alterations of bodies, τὴν τροπὴν τῶν σωμάτων. Despite the impressiveness of this terminology, it does not turn up elsewhere, but appears to be rhetorically effective coinages by the author himself.

It is probably true, then, as people have argued, that the first two letters, which tie the king's invitation to a Persian plague, were composed later than, and, rather cleverly, as an introduction to, the letters that follow. The case seems strengthened by the fact that the ancient papyrus manuscripts of the letters contain only letters 3-6 and 11 (and the epistolographic manuscript Parisinus graecus 3052 contains only 3-9). There are grounds for asking whether the manuscript tradition can offer insight into the dates at which the letters were composed.

---

[50] The name is discussed by Dimitrios Th. Sakalis, "Beiträge zu den pseudo-hippokratischen Briefen." in *Formes de pensée dans la collection hippocratique*, ed. F. Lasserre and P. Mudry. (Geneva:1983) pp. 504-5. Though the rest of Sakalis' argument about the purpose of the letters is rather unfortunate, his proposal that the addressee of Artaxerxes' letter is an Oriental is eminently reasonable.

One notes that letters 3-6 and also 11, which is their companion in the papyrus texts, concentrate on the ways in which venality harms the science, selecting that theme out of the potentially more complex dramas. But, in fact, letter 11 does mention a Persian plague, and that suggests that it was written after the substance, at least, of letter 1 existed, and thus seems to me to defeat the arguments of those who insist that letter 1 must have been written after the date of the papyri because 3-6 are unaware of the plague.

Further, 7-9 do not appear in the papyrus manuscripts, which is the only thing that might lead one to distinguish them from the others. They match 3-6 in style and tone. 7 is a letter of transmittal, perhaps with a pun on a Persian name, that, like 3-6, shows how intriguing the author found the process of getting letters to and from a Persian king. 8 is a handsome letter which uses intemperate language and concludes that Hippocrates has a bad character because he rejected the invitation. Letter 9 comes up to 8 in quality, affecting Coan dialect and characterizing the brave independence of the populace of the small island. The economy, or reticence, of the writing in 7-9 incline me to associate them closely with 3-6, and I infer that they were simply omitted from some selections. I conclude that our papyrus manuscripts exhibit a brief selection from the whole, and that they cannot tell us about the assembly of the whole collection. This conclusion affects our estimate of letter 11 in its relation to the Democritus group of letters: it, too, is pulled from a larger group.

One is still left with the question of sequence of composition. The whole group including 1 and 2 is more interesting literarily than letters 3 and following by themselves, a fact which in itself provides motive for their composition. Letter 2's celebration of Hippocrates' genealogy, and its exploration of the notion that he changed the nature of the medical profession tells us more of the author's interests, and I would infer from his creative medical terminology that the author of 1-2 is an intellectual, non-physician. The author's statement that the Athenians and others sanctified Hippocrates and worshiped him in his lifetime removes it from the speeches and *Decree*, which are presumably its sources. Does the name Paetus tell us anything, or to put it another way, how useful is the conjecture that names of correspondents of 1-2 and other letters were chosen to flatter people who bore those names and were contemporary with the author of the letters? It is a good academic idea, the sort of idea which once proposed resists testing, and is fruitful of endless conjectures.[51]

---

[51] J. F. Marcks, *Symbolae Criticae* (Diss, Bonn: 1883), has been influential, in the absence of competing interpretations, in dating all the collections to the same period in Rome. He had two arguments (p. 43-4) about names in the Hippocratic letters: that there must have been a Crateuas, grandson of Mithridates, whom letter 16 was intended to flatter, and that the name Dionysius must be used in order to flatter Dionysius of Halicarnassus. Subsequently Diels used flattery of contemporaries as a general principle for dating the letters in *Hippocratische Forschungen V*, *Hermes* 53 (1918) 57-87, and found a Paetus of the second century A.D. Philippson dated the letters to 44 B.C. by finding a different, earlier Paetus: Robert Philippson, "Verfasser und Abfassungzeit der sogennante Hippokrates-briefe" *Rheinisches Museum* 77 (1928) 293-328. Fridolf Kudlien developed Diels's conjecture further in the article "Paetus", in RE Suppl. 10

The Democritus Letters

Letters 10-17

The novella in letters which relates to Hippocrates' visit to Democritus expands some minimal biographical conjectures: Hippocrates and Democritus were contemporaries, and therefore must have known one another. Material for the expansion, as it relates to Democritus, is provided by moral philosophy, largely cynic-stoic, which dramatizes the superior, cultured wise man in his relations to society. As it relates to Hippocrates, material for expansion is provided, so far as one can see, not by historical information, but by the current sense of the medical profession, which creates for Hippocrates a personality fit for the successful medical man as conceived by the writers. That more than one writer is involved seems clear from the way the letters after 17 differ from 10-17. Modern readers, especially in the nineteenth century, have been put off by this father of medicine, who, when he invents the *techne*, is not an aloof scientist formulating scientific method for medicine and promoting intellectual or other revolution, but a practical organizer, self-conscious, indeed, about ethical aspects of his craft and about the serious issues raised by questions of what is normal and abnormal. This Hippocrates knows the proper place of a wife, the value of friendship, the socially destructive effects of greed, and the emotional volatility of mobs. But his perspective is imperfect before he comes to know the sage Democritus, who can give insight into the utter pettiness of most human concerns. The added letters, 18-21, introduce other ideas. We can consider their

---

(1965) 473-4. Sakalis' proposal (n. 50) is a needed corrective. To take such dating of the letters by the name Paetus seriously we have to be convinced that a Paetus would feel honored to be figured as the correspondent of the Persian king who had received many presents, and that producers and users of the Hippocratic Corpus and the bibliographic material attached to it would engage in and enjoy this kind of falsification as part of their experience of Hippocratic material. I have not seen any discussion that faces that question directly. The inference about the name Krateuas is still more tortured: Hippocrates addresses a Krateuas in Letter 16, and says that he is as good as his προπάτωρ. Marcks begged all intervening questions and invented a grandson of the famous Krateuas, physician to Mithridates VI, who died in 63 B.C., to be the object of flattery. But Diels and others who have subscribed to the notion (e.g., Kind in RE s.v. Krateuas), were apparently unaware that Alexis, a fourth-third century comic poet wrote a Κρατεύας ἢ Φαρμακοπώλης. The letter can readily refer to a historical or imagined person contemporary with or older than Hippocrates, and need not involve a jarring anachronistic violation of the dramatic date of the letter. True, the comic figure, Krateuas the drug-vender, was probably not presented as a dignified intellectual, but quite the contrary (See R. Morel, s.v. Pharmakopoles, RE 19 pt. 2 [1939] cols. 1840-1). Nonetheless, my argument is that in order to satisfy the conceit of the Hippocratic letter, one needs only a sense of the figure of Crateuas and the sense of family tradition.

dating and the relation between the groups after considering the substance of the whole.

Letter 17

The seventeenth letter provides the climax and the intellectual center of the novella, bringing its themes to fruition. Dramatically, the letter maintains its narrative point of view precisely and with good effect. Hippocrates, the narrator, describes himself as competent and optimistic, ready to calm the frightened and over-emotional Abderites and to face the problem of madness if it exists. His narrative of the walk to Democritus' house and of the setting in which Democritus is studying is told in an objective way, but its language evokes symbolism that pastoral poetry and philosophy had developed, the pale and emaciated, hermit-like philosopher, the babbling brook and spreading trees of the rural retreat, and even a sanctuary of the nymphs, the sort of place where something extraordinary and supernatural will happen to those who are open to it.[52]

When the two men meet, Democritus' courtesy and apparent sanity disarm the narrator. He is also, apparently, sincerely impressed by Democritus' assiduous anatomical research on animal carcasses. Democritus seeks the gall, "its nature and place," because its excess or deficiency is conceived as the source of madness as well as of other disease. The effect of this would depend on when it was written and what views were current about anatomical research, as we shall note below. In response, instead of referring to his own comparable investigations, Hippocrates wishes he had leisure to do some research, and is brought up short when Democritus laughs violently at his expression of regret that his numerous mundane concerns prevent him from having time to investigate the nature of things. Hippocrates gently reproves Democritus for his excessive and inappropriate laughter, and offers to cure him of his affection or to undergo

---

[52] There appears to be here a reminiscence of Plato, *Phaedrus*, 230.b, where Socrates describes the setting of the dialogue in a place sacred to the nymphs. Νὴ τὴν Ἥραν, καλή γε ἡ καταγωγή. ἥ τε γὰρ πλάτανος αὕτη μάλ' ἀμφιλαφής τε καὶ ὑψηλή. However, the phrases became commonplace after Plato used them, if they were not earlier. Compare similar settings in Euripides' *Hippolytus* and the epigram by Thyillus of the first century B.C.

πῶς ἂν δροσερᾶς ἀπὸ κρηνῖδος
καθαρῶν ὑδάτων πῶμ' ἀρυσαίμαν,
ὑπό τ' αἰγείροις ἔν τε κομήτῃ
λειμῶνι κλιθεῖσ' ἀναπαυσαίμαν ;
(Phaedra at *Hippolytus* 209ff)

Αἱ πτελέαι τῷ Πανὶ καὶ αἱ τανυμήκεες αὗται
ἰτέαι ἥ θ' ἱερὰ κἀμφιλαφὴς πλάτανος
καὶ λιβάδες καὶ ταῦτα βοτηρικὰ Πανὶ κύπελλα
ἄγκειται, δίψης φάρμακ' ἀλεξίκακα.
(Anth. Pal. 6.170)

correction himself, and he goes straight to the point: sanity requires making distinctions between good and bad. Democritus in turn offers his own therapy, the picture of humans wasting their lives on valueless activities worthy only of laughter. Hippocrates' ironic reply is wasted on him: Perhaps the whole world is ill and has nowhere to go for therapy, for what is outside it? He is told that there is an infinity of worlds, and that he should not belittle nature's riches. Democritus' first wave of description of irrational human behavior does not do its job. Hippocrates still can claim that there are objects inappropriate for laughter. People strive because they must, necessity drives them to choice and action, and they cannot help it if they go wrong. Democritus' second wave of description is more analytical, employing terms developed by Cynics, Stoics and Epicureans to signal mental and moral instability which the philosophies aim at curing, but there is apparent Democritean language also in the description of life as change. Failure to use the senses, to recognize their own limitations, and to adjust their desires to reality, insures the mindless vacillation that Democritus laughs at in men. This second wave terminates in another extended list of human irrationalities which seems to get out of hand and become repetitious. One may suspect that it has been extended by additions after the original composition.

The narrative ends abruptly with Hippocrates' sudden conversion to Democritus' point of view, and that conversion is presented without the qualifying wit that one might desire. And, as Temkin points out, the cynic laughter of the ending leaves us unresolved as to the proposed nature of medical science: what would a humane Cynical science do?[53] One literary effect, somewhat grotesque, but too compelling to ignore, is probably present in the ending: Hippocrates says that he will become Democritus' herald, κῆρυξ. Athenaeus[54] preserves from Machaon's reminiscences of the wandering musician Stratonicus this joke: Stratonicus went to Abdera and found that each Abderite had his own herald, κῆρυξ, through whom he could proclaim when he wanted the coming of the new moon. As a result, there were in Abdera more heralds than citizens. Stratonicus, when asked why he was walking on tiptoes, said that he did so for fear that he would step on a κῆρυξ (either "herald", or the shell of a whelk or limpet), and ruin his foot. If the audience is supposed to recall that story about Abdera, the author is thumbing his nose somewhat at the audience's engagement in the more serious questions he has suggested, and this certainly affects our response as audience. We should also acknowledge another, subtle, literary effect at this point. In Letter 15, the goddess Truth told Hippocrates that he would find her at Democritus' house. Now, at the end of Letter 17, without specific language to recall the earlier letter, Hippocrates sees Democritus as virtually a god whose wisdom will teach men σωφρονίζειν, "to be reasonable and decent." He

---

[53] Owsei Temkin, "Hippocrates as the Physician of Democritus," *Gesnerus* 42 (1985) 455-464, esp. 461-2.

[54] *Deipnosophistae* 8.349 b. Also in A. S. F. Gow, ed., *Machaon*, Cambridge Classical Texts and Commentaries (Cambridge: 1965) p. 41.

promises that he will come back the following days for further instruction, and then will go forth as the herald of Democritus' wisdom. He announces to the "true Abderites" what he has learned. We may notice another touch at the end: a servant silently appears to receive the books of Democritus when he rises from his seat. This perhaps surprises us if we have started thinking of Democritus as a mendicant Cynic. We have to adjust our response, and to think of Democritus more as an eccentric aristocrat on his country estate than as a hermit.

10-16

Letters 10-16, which set the scene for Hippocrates' encounter with Democritus have comparable touches of comedy of manners which enhance the novella's effect. The strokes are often broad, but there are subtle ones as well. The Abderites' appeal is properly hysterical and insensitive (particularly about money); Hippocrates is properly cautious about diagnosis but ready to make great exertions in the humane task.[55] In letter 12, in which he accepts an offer of entertainment in Abdera, he begins the development of psychological ideas with a brief discourse on the nature of melancholy, a discourse whose terms recall Aristotle, *Problems* 30.1, the classic text on the subject in antiquity,[56] but considers other possibilities as well, finally foreshadowing what the actual event will show. In letter 13, in which he enlists a friend to come to watch over his affairs in his absence, he manages a lecture on the nature of women and the proper control of them. In 14, while requesting a ship for transportation, he takes seriously the notion that a melancholic Democritus is truly out of bounds in his scorn of the world. Letter 15, on his dream of Asclepius, shows Hippocrates as the sensitive, pious man who is specially guided by the god. In 16, requesting drugs from his root cutter, he discourses on the evil of greed and offers a lecture on pharmacology. These letters show the double competence of the great scientific intellect, as Hippocrates organizes his mundane affairs efficiently. When, finally, Hippocrates receives the therapy for his διανοίη in letter 17, after confessing that his success in mundane affairs robs him of the time to think, the details of these earlier letters are cast into a new light. The result is a rather pleasing literary structure. The letters preceding 17 can only be thought to be accretions if one fails to see the pretty structure of the group.[57] Perhaps letter 11, the response to the Abderites, stands out. It has some especially turgid language, e.g., "I am persuaded that science is the gift of the gods" (πειθόμενος). I was convinced (as was the case) that the matter was pressing πεισθείς, ὅπερ ἦν, ἐπε ίγειν τὸ πρῆγμα, but it has nothing that is incompatible with the

[55] Owsei Temkin (n. 53) describes well the considerations of differential diagnosis involved in Hippocrates' musings, p. 456-7.

[56] Jackie Pigeaud, in *La maladie de l' âme* (Paris: 1981) pp. 452-477, offers a sensitive reading of the Democritus letters in reference to the theme of madness and its cure by laughter.

[57] Edelstein, for example, said that the letter to Krateuas is "inorganic". The plot does not depend on it in any way. But that is simply to take an odd view of what the letters are about.

characterization of Hippocrates in the rest of the group. 11 is in the papyrus manuscripts, possibly alone, and in the epistolographic tradition in manuscripts in which 10-17 occur without 18ff, a fact that might incline us to think that the collection grew by accretion around 11, or that 10 was written later than the rest. But 11 could have been selected from the larger collection for the papyrus selection as representing important sentiments from the mouth of Hippocrates. It contains a serious expression of medical ethics regarding money: who hires out prostitutes his *techne*, which is also the theme in the selected group of Persian letters. Hippocrates' diatribe on passions as diseases of the soul which is embedded in 11's lecture on money is also classic, having a Stoic ring. Letter 11 embodies in brief the story of Artaxerxes' invitation, and it gives the impressive description of the festival of the renewal of the staff in Cos.[58] We should recognize the possibility that Letter 11 can stand alone, and could have provided a core around which the other letters were composed. My own feeling is that letter 10 is detachable, though well composed for the group, and that occurrences and non-occurrences in the manuscript tradition are more suggestive in its case that it is not part of the original group.

Democritus' investigation of the animal gall-bladder and bile in Letter 17 is not modelled on any known investigation in antiquity. For writer and intended audience, the investigation shows Democritus' seriousness and sophistication, and casts Hippocrates in the light of a naif. In describing the premises of his study, Democritus says that παρακοπή is for the most part caused by excessive bile; bile is by nature present in all, some more, some less, and diseases are its ἀμετρίη, its excess; bile is a material sometimes good, sometimes bad.

"Diseases are its excess" is the letter writer's own formulation. The term ἀμετρίη, or ἀμετρία, is used in medical writings of the Hellenistic period and later, usually in reference to environmental factors, never of the bile. In non-medical writers it is in common use from the fifth century on in moral contexts, similar to its thematic use in the Democritus sequence of letters to refer to Democritus' condition. In the 13th letter Hippocrates muses that what Democritus suffers may not be a disease but ἀμετρίη παιδείης, an excess of learning, culture, study, thought to be excess by laymen, but not really so, since excess of virtue is never a bad thing. Again in Letter 14, Hippocrates plans to reprove Democritus for his ἀμετρίη. In Democritus' diatribe in Letter 17 he speaks of human failings as ἄμετροι ἐπιθυμίαι and ὀργὴ ἀμέτρος. We need not look to medicine for the source of the term Democritus uses, then, but we note that the phrase ὀργὴ ἀμέτρος is reminiscent of a sentiment actually expressed by the historical Democritus, κακὰ πάντα παρακολουθεῖ διὰ τὰς ὑπερμέτρους

---

[58] An interesting ceremony is described at the opening of 11, the analepsis of the rhabdos, presumably the renewal of the staff of the statue of Asclepius, a ceremony which is not described elsewhere. Is it an invention of the author on the pattern of a ceremony elsewhere, or does it, as Sherwin White (*Ancient Cos* 340-341) says, assure us that there really was such a ceremony?

ὀργάς, "all evils come in the wake of excessive passions."[59] We will return to this below.

The statement "Bile is sometimes good and sometimes bad" seems also to be original with the letter writer. One will search long for a similar view in the medical writings. Bile is in the Hippocratic Corpus generally a cause of disease, particularly of fever. *Diseases 1*.2 can be taken as the normal view: the internal factors that cause disease are bile and phlegm, which are always present in some amount, but food, drink, or environmental factors can make them produce disease. In *Sacred Disease* the bile is responsible for one kind of madness (the term there is μαινόμενοι, παρακοπή is not used): "Those maddened by bile are noisy, make trouble, and are restless, always doing something inappropriate."[60] The *Sacred Disease* does not ascribe the affection to the gall bladder, though it describes at length the anatomy of the other kind of madness, from phlegm. Aristotle discussed the existence and place of the gall bladder in *Parts of Animals* Book 4, ch. 2. His concern in that work is to show Nature's providence, and to find the purpose for all things. But his creativity fails in the face of the gall and the gall bladder. He has to conclude that not everything is for a purpose; some things are for a necessity that is created by things which are for a purpose, and such is the gall.[61] Athenaeus managed to make fun of Aristotle because of his fascination with which animal had and which did not have a gall bladder.[62] Mnesitheus of Athens denied that the elephant had a gall bladder, and Galen corrected him.[63] But Galen is reticent on the subject of the purpose of the gall, and indeed I cannot parallel the assertion of Letter 17. The reason is that no one imagined that the bile was useful in digestion, nor could anyone conceive another use. Aristotle's view is the standard one. Use of the term ὕλη, substance or matter, in the description of bile by the author of Letter 17 suggests both that the letter is post-Aristotelian and that an elemental theory lurks behind the formulation, even though one would not look for an elemental constituent in one place in the body, only a pathological one. This suggests some influence from the view expressed in *Nature of Man* in the Hippocratic Corpus, that yellow and black bile are normal constituents of the human body (in that sense they could be called good, though the Hippocratic author does not so call them), whose seasonal increase and excess cause diseases. The author of *Nature of Man*, aside from his elemental theory, has normal views, as shown in his section on the fevers that bile causes.[64] He himself would not have said what Democritus says in Letter 17, nor sought understanding in Democritus' manner, but he is in the background of what is said.

---

[59] D-K frag. B 143, from Philodemus *De ira*.

[60] οἱ δὲ ὑπὸ χολῆς κεκράκται τε καὶ κακοῦργοι καὶ οὐκ ἀτρεμαῖοι, ἀλλ' αἰεί τι ἄκαιρον δρῶντες.

[61] *De Partibus Animalium* , 676 b16-677 b14.

[62] *Deipnosophistae* 8.353 d-e, in reference to Aristotle, *HA* 506.

[63] *Anat. Admin.*, Kühn 2.69.

[64] Chapter 15, Littré 6.66-8. For its close relation to the earlier part see the discussion by Jacques Jouanna in his edition, CMG 1.1.3 (Berlin: 1975) 22-34.

Democritus investigates madness by investigating its seat, an activity that seems simple and straightforward to us, and did to later antiquity, but is too sophisticated for the period that provides the dramatic date of the letter, and probably before the first century B.C. The idea of the affected place as the cause of disease is normal in Greek medicine from the earliest material that we have, as witness *Sacred Disease's* confidence that the epileptic goat's head will be found to be full of water,[65] and the numerous descriptions of the conditions of the interior of the body imagined to account for symptoms. *Ancient Medicine* proposes relating textures and shapes of organs to perceived symptoms,[66] but systematic study of the specific relations of organs, in their size, shape and condition, to normal and pathological phenomena came somewhat later, out of the work of the anatomists of Alexandria. Aristotle's investigations of organs in the *Parts of Animals* are a search for ἀρχαί, for the sources and causes of their presence or absence in the various animals, and for their normal function, with an eye to classification of animals and man into higher and lower, less and more perfect. Implications for pathological anatomy are there, but are not pursued. Diocles' anatomy, of which we know little beyond its being the first that Galen knew, asks whether the body has this or that part, what is the shape of the uterus, etc., in the preserved fragments.[67] Diocles' pathological work, in *Affection, Cause, Treatment*, relates affection to organs in the Hippocratic manner, to imagined malfunction, irritation, blockage.[68] It was Herophilus and Erasistratus who opened bodies to attempt to correlate shape, size and conditions of organs with normal and pathological phenomena, as Democritus is apparently doing. They used human subjects, and were, if Galen is accurate, effectively without successors before Marinus revived their pursuits using animals for dissection and study.[69] We would place Marinus in the first-second century A.D. The writer of Letter 17 is not necessarily writing in the wake of Marinus. He could have come up with the notion of Democritus' research himself or have been stimulated by others' musings on the subject before Marinus. But I think that the subject would not have occurred to him as it did before the time of Herophilus, and probably not for some time later until the anatomy was generally known. The author shows no signs of being a physician.[70]

---

[65] *Sacred Disease*, Littré 6.382.

[66] *Ancient Medicine*, ch. 22, Littré 1.626-634.

[67] Diocles' *Anatomy* is fragments 23-29 in Wellmann's collection: Max Wellmann, *Die Fragmente der sikilischen Aerzte Akron, Philistion, und des Diokles von Karystos*, (Berlin: 1901).

[68] Diocles Fragments 37-82, Wellmann.

[69] In his description of his own epitomies of Marinus' work, Galen tells us that Marinus dealt with the liver, and the gall bladder which is on the liver in the twelfth book of his work, which was a combined anatomy and physiology. Galen, *On his own Books*, *Scr. min.* 2, 107 (ed., Iwan Müller).

[70] Simplistic answers to questions of the author's training and outlook should be avoided, such as Philippson's statement that the author is of course a rhetor, and Celsus, too, was a rhetor, so dabbling in medicine is no indication of being a physician (n. 51 above, p. 309); the other

We need further to belabor the bit of humor created by the author of Letter 17, by asking what general view of Hippocrates the author expected his audience to have, i.e., how they would receive Hippocrates' plaintive wish that he had time to do research in the interior of the body. I have mentioned earlier Galen's arguments in his *Anatomical Procedures* that Hippocrates knew all of medicine including anatomy, but transmitted it orally. Galen is original and overexuberant in his Hippocratic interpretations in that direction, and he did not have predecessors who made such extreme claims. But there are hints of discussions in the Hellenistic period in which Hippocrates was put forward as one who, in Celsus' terms, pursued the Nature of Things. When Celsus describes disputes between Empirics and Dogmatics about knowledge of causes, and, in relation to that, about the importance of anatomy, he tells us that the Dogmatics had claimed Hippocrates as their predecessor. Celsus' discussion lacks detail about who said what when, but he reflects generations of discussion when he says,

> It is probable that Hippocrates, Erasistratus, and certain others, who were not content to busy themselves over fevers and ulcerations, but also to some extent searched into the nature of things, did not by this become physicians, but became by it greater physicians.[71]

Celsus, incidentally, also says that Hippocrates, according to some, was a student of Democritus.[72] It seems probable that Celsus thus acknowledges Letter 17, or some reflection of it. The wit of Letter 17 reflects serious discussions and assertions about the nature of medical thought and development of method. But it does so in a distorted way: Democritus' doctrine in Letter 17 is not about medical thought and method, it is about the philosophic life, with some incidental suggestion, in the manner of Socrates, that if you choose the philosophic life all else follows. We note, however, that what follows in this case reflects discussions about medicine of the period after about 200 B.C.

We now proceed to the aspect of Letter 17 that has received the most attention, and on the basis of which it is usually judged and dated. Democritus' speech belongs to a recognizable literary genre, the diatribe, which in its developed form discourses with more or less wit and indignation the follies and vices of mankind in imitation of Diogenes and the other cynics. Roman Satire developed an elegant version of it, apparently with some influence from the Cynic Menippus, of the early third century B.C. Not only has the work of Menippus almost

---

extreme is offered by Sakalis (n. 50 above) p. 501, who proves that the author is a physician by quoting statements that show general interest in medicine.

[71] Celsus, *De Medicina*, Proemium 47 (ed. Marx): Verique simile est et Hippocratem et Erasistratum, et quicumque alii non contenti febres et ulcera agitare rerum quoque naturam aliqua parte scrutati sunt, non ideo quidem medicos fuisse, verum ideo quoque maiores medicos extitisse.

[72] Proemium 8. For a discussion of Celsus' point of view about Hippocrates, see *The Hippocratic Tradition*, pp. 225-30.

totally perished, but so has the rest of early Cynic literature. Diogenes of Sinope founded the Cynic tradition in the early fourth century, and was seconded by Crates who spread his philosophy.[73] He himself probably established the values to which the Cynics ascribed and the terminology for them, which were passed down in sayings, anecdotes, and diatribes. The values included αὐτάρκεια, self-sufficiency, and ἀναίδεια, shamelessness. Shamelessness involved flouting conventional manners and morality and living in the natural way. Indeed, Diogenes was said to have accepted the comparison to the behavior of dogs, which gave the sect its name. Crates wrote letters which embodied Cynic views and which were much praised (though the letters preserved under his name are not the genuine ones). The Cynics also promoted παιδεία and δικαιοσύνη. Their tendencies are related to the philosophical traditions of various sorts that traced their origins back to Socrates. The tradition of Cynic letters, then, stems from as early as the last part of the fourth century. But that early material is lost, and the letters we have in the names of the major Cynics seem to come from somewhat later and to be epistolographic dramatizations of the Cynic biographies of the sort that we find in Diogenes Laertius book 6. None of the preserved letters can be dated precisely, but the tendency of scholars has been to date the genre as a whole to the last century B.C and the first and second A.D., in part on the inference that the Cynic tradition died out in the second century and was revived in a new, Stoic form only in the first century. Adjustments to those views remain to be made in the light of Dudley's arguments that the Cynic tradition did not die and experience rebirth, but was continuous. Increasing work on and interest in the epistolographic material promises some revaluation, or more convincing affirmation.

The Hippocratic letters 10-17 do not put themselves in the same category as the Cynic letters but are more refined. They do not set out to rub the reader's nose in a doctrine, nor to engage in a leveling disparagement of major philosophies. True, Democritus' guffaws at the shallowness of his townsmen constitute a breach of the decorum they expect, but the effect is very different from that of Diogenes' breaches of decorum by pointed insult, or more dramatically by public masturbation or by spitting in his host's face, or by recommending stealing from temples. In the Hippocratic letters, mild, uplifting sentiments are set forth in a dramatic context of normalcy and courtesy, and Democritus has only a few of the trappings of the mendicant saint, more like Socrates than Diogenes. Yet the Hippocratic letters do not approach the level of seriousness and concern with genuine philosophic issues that the letters of the minor Socratics and of Plato do. The laughing Democritus acknowledges, especially with his diatribe, the Cynic view.

Zeph Stewart presents interesting and convincing arguments that the ethical sayings of Democritus, which turn up in the florilegia and make up a large

---

[73] I follow here the account of D. R. Dudley, *A History of Cynicism* (London: 1937).

proportion of the fragments, were selected and preserved in a Cynic tradition.[74] In an attempt to date the laughing Democritus as an invention of that tradition, Stewart is led to the circle of Menippus.[75] The themes of the Hippocratic letters, Democritus' laughter, and the stupid Abderites are first used by Cicero,[76] who, of course, did not invent them. Nothing gets us any closer to the specific date of the Democritus sequence, which could have been written any time in the two centuries before the first century papyrus which testifies that Letter 11 was read in Egypt in the early first century A.D., and it could have been written in the eastern or western Mediterranean.

The letters of Heraclitus show a number of parallels with those of Hippocrates.[77] Heraclitus in Letter 1 is invited by Darius to be given wealth and honor as a guest in Persia. He refuses, not out of patriotism, but because it is appropriate to live on little. He is threatened, as his seventh letter says, by an Ephesian law that would exile all misanthropes, and those who do not laugh. He explains that he does not laugh because he hates man's wickedness, evidence of which he details: fraud, lust, war, gluttony, luxury. And he compares beasts favorably with mankind, exactly the themes that Democritus develops to explain his laughter. The seventh letter, which contains Heraclitus' diatribe appears to have been subject to expansion by the addition of indignant detail. Thus, in a second century A.D. version recovered in a papyrus (P. Gen. 271), Heraclitus goes on from the point at which the medieval manuscripts end, to add further comparisons of man with animals and to denounce poets for their portrayals of immorality.[78] But despite generic similarity between the Hippocratic and Heraclitean letters, there are no obvious verbal connections. The Heraclitean letters are, like the Cynic letters generally, very insulting about the medical profession. In letters 5 and 6, Heraclitus says that the physicians cannot understand dropsy and cannot cure it, because they cannot turn a rainstorm into a drought. Far from knowing and imitating the cosmos as the way to healing, the doctors simply massaged him like a leather bottle. But doctors had killed his uncle, Heracleodorus, and pocketed the reward. The Heraclitean letters are plausibly dated to the first century B.C.[79]

---

[74] "Democritus and the Cynics," *Harvard Studies in Classical Philology* 63 (1958) 179-191. For a recent evaluation of the ethical fragments, see Charles Kahn, "Democritus and the Origins of Moral Psychology," *AJP* 106 (1985) 1-31.

[75] pp. 185-6.

[76] *De Oratore* 2.58.235 for the laughter, *Att.* 4.16 and 7.7 for the stupidity of Abderites. Horace, *Epist.* 2.1.194-200 uses the theme of the laughter, and Juvenal, 10.34 and 46-53 uses both themes.

[77] Available (text, translation, introduction) in Harold W. Attridge, *First Century Cynicism in the Epistles of Heraclitus* (Scholars Press, Missoula, Montana: 1976) .

[78] Published by V. Martin, "Une recueil de diatribes cyniques: Pap. Gen. 271," *Museum Helveticum* 16 (1969) 77-117. There has been some disagreement as to whether the papyrus represents an original or an expanded version of the Heraclitean letter. I follow Leonardo Taran: R. Mondolfo and L. Taran, *Eraclito, Testimonianze e Imitazioni*, (Florence: 1972) 298. The other view is expressed by Attridge, pp. 8-11.

[79] Discussed by Attridge (n. 77) pp. 5-6.

18-21

The group 18-21 are written from a different point of view than the group 10-17. 18 does not commence from the tone of the conversion in 17, though the basic facts addressed are the same, save for what Democritus was employed in thinking about when Hippocrates arrived. This Democritus is rather annoyed in 18 at the danger Hippocrates posed for him, carrying the dangerous drug hellebore around, ready to use it in therapy. He writes on the physician's need for thoughtfulness and adduces terms from his philosophy to validate his credentials: Democritus has found the nature of reality and separated it from the ἰνδαλμοί, the wandering motes, or perhaps images, that confuse our vision. The medical man, too, he writes, must judge from reality (πρῆγμα), not the undependable sense of sight, must know the configurations (ῥυθμοί), and treat the totality of the body (σκῆνος), not just the πάθος. He sends a treatise on madness, a treatise he calls his own, which is made out of excerpts from *Sacred Disease*.

How, one asks, could this letter be so near to the substance of 17 and yet so discrepant? It is possible that 17 and 18-19 are independent versions of the story of Hippocrates' visit to Democritus, neither writer aware of the other, or that one was written in as an alternative to or "correction" of the other. Different views on this subject have been held without conclusive arguments being advanced, and the discussion has been complicated by other matters. Hermann Diels considered the discrepancies insignificant and attributed 1-24 to the same author, arguing against the view of Marcks that they were by separate authors.[80] Diels was much moved by what he took to be a longer, altered version of letter 19 that appears in a sixteenth century manuscript, Urbinas graecus 68. Diels was taken by a notion that Max Pohlenz had put forward, that in the papyri we had original editions and second editions of some letters by the author himself.[81] He concluded that the treatise on rabies in Urb. 68, which is much longer than Letter 19, but uses some of the same material in the midst of a pastiche of Hippocratic and other medical works, was a second edition of Letter 19 by the same author. I suspect that the attraction of that conclusion, along with his general contempt for the letters, led him to assert that the letters, however discrepant, were all the product of one hand. Philippson[82] supported the notion. Hans Diller pointed out some time later that the treatise on rabies is added to the text of Urb. 68, and is a sixteenth century forgery, or perhaps one should say exercise.[83] Edelstein, and so far as I know, everyone else, has since thought that 18-21 are by a different

---

[80] H. Diels, *Hermes* 53 (1918) 84, who discusses Marcks, *Symbola Critica ad Epistolographos graecos* (Bonn) 1883.
[81] Max Pohlenz, "Zu den hippokratischen Briefen," *Hermes* 52 (1917) 348-353.
[82] Cited in n. 51 above.
[83] Hans Diller, "Die sogennante zweite Fassung des 19. Hippokratesbriefes," *Quellen und Studien zur Geschichte der Naturwissenschaften und der Medizin* III.4 (1933) 35-44.

author or authors than the preceding ones.[84] Recently, Herman De Ley has argued that there is a strong contradiction between the two presentations of the meeting of Hippocrates and Democritus.[85] He reads letters 18-21 as anti-Hippocratic, and conjectures that letters 1-17 were written to counter their effect. He is forced to conjecture also that the author of 1-17 was constrained not to contradict the tradition that 18-21 represent, while making Hippocrates more respectable and less absurd, and that subsequently, he must conjecture, the two groups were combined into one by happenstance.[86] In my view De Ley overstates the abusiveness of letter 18, which in any case is moderated by the reply of 20. Democritus' suspicions of Hippocrates are exaggerated, as patients' suspicions sometimes are. The author of this group does not descend to having Hippocrates say "I have never given medicine inappropriately," or "I am, after all, the sainted Hippocrates." Instead, he has him respond that mistakes are possible. The reader is aware that no mistake was made in this instance. And there are no grounds for saying that 1-17 respond specifically to 18-21. In addition, De Ley conjectures that the author of 18-21 was actually confused about the authorship of the *Sacred Disease*, and that of the *Epidemics*, and he argues that that confusion is evidence that Letters 18-21 were written early, before the *Corpus* was known. That seems to me to be a counsel of desperation. The kind of confusion involved in attributing those works to Democritus is unlikely at any time. On the other hand, it is an odd witticism to attribute *Sacred Disease* to Democritus in order to produce a treatise on madness for him, but that is apparently what the author of 19 has done, meanwhile acknowledging Hippocrates' *Epidemics* and quoting them back to him. Knowledge of the corpora of the two great men is part of the point of 18-21. The author plays with known texts of Democritus and Hippocrates while dealing, in a dilettant's manner, with technical and ethical issues that they raise. As we noticed above, 10-17, which have their own brand of moralizing, are not close to the specific work of the great men, but move in an atmosphere of commonplace and abstraction.

So, assuming that the two groups are by different authors, it is easily possible that they are independent of one another, two versions of a story that was current about Hippocrates and the "mad" Democritus, but I think it more likely that the notion of the treatise on madness comes to Letter 18 from 17, but that the author of 18-21, while getting inspiration from 17, is less interested in the Cynic drama of conversion than he is in the literary possibility of an exchange and challenge between two wise men, of whose work he knows something. If the author of 18-21 took the idea of the treatise on madness from 17, as I suspect, he dropped the notion that it was a treatise on the nature and place of the gall, because no such

---

[84] Edelstein's discussion is in RE Supp. 6 (1935) col. 1204-5.

[85] Herman De Ley, *De samenstelling van de Pseudo-Hippokratische Brievenversameling en haar plaats in de traditie. Handelingen der Kon. Zuidnederlandse Mats. voor Taal- en Letterkunde en Geschiedenis*, XXIII (1969) 47-80.

[86] De Ley 78-9

treatise was available to him from anywhere. But he could make a treatise by borrowing from *Sacred Disease*, as he did.

Letter 19 begins with an explanation of madness that is Hippocratic in its physiology, Democritean in its epistemology: excessive moisture in the brain distorts perception, and what the tongue of the madman speaks is what the distorted perception is receiving. The rest is from *Sacred Disease* and *Epidemics 5*.

Letter 20, Hippocrates' own cover letter for a treatise on hellebore, commences with a commonplace about common failure to appreciate medicine,[87] but he admits that his medicine has not reached perfection, nor did that of Asclepius before him, as one can infer from transmitted writings. He then answers mildly to Democritus' criticism of his actions and transmits his treatise on treatment with hellebore. One is naturally curious whether the author of these letters made the compilation himself. Excerpt literature is the stuff of medicine, and *Aphorisms*, from which the core of the treatise comes, is already excerpt literature which physicians would adapt and expand for their own purposes. Because hellebore is so dangerous, but remained prominent as a remedy, everyone would naturally try to be up to date on it.

The Miscellaneous Letters 22-24

The Letters 22-24 do not belong to the other groups. 22, recommending geometry to Thessalos, stands apart, 23 is a literary exercise on anatomy, and 24 appears to refer to 23, or to another work like it, and to to be an introduction to a Regimen. All three letters subscribe to the notion of medicine as *paideia*. Where and when they became part of the collection is not clear, but some conjectures, at least, can be ruled out.

Letter 23 has a detachable philosophic dietetic proem, which does not fit the subject matter of the letter itself but reads as though it was written when 23 was made part of the collection. That is to say, I suspect that the person responsible for this letter borrowed the anatomy and composed the proem. He recommends medicine for two reasons: because it is good for those engaged with literature and culture in general, and because medicine keeps one healthy and keeps the body from interfering in intellectual pursuits. One must anticipate disease, which develops even during health, for disease will weaken the body's will to pursue virtue. One is reminded of Celsus' observation that philosophers busied themselves with medicine because mental activity is so hard on the body, and also one is reminded of Erotian's observation that Hippocrates is worth reading for anyone interested in λογικὴ παιδεῖα (literary culture), by which he means

[87]Similar statements can be found in the Hippocratic Corpus, e.g., *De arte* ch. 4 (Li. 6.6), *Dis. 1*, ch. 8 (Li. 6.156).

particularly the history of the Greek language.[88] The anatomy in 23 is not going to keep anyone healthy, of course. Its tone and purpose are summed up near the end: it describes the different types of organs that have been designed for use by an incorporeal nature resident in the inner sanctums of the body. The anatomy simply names the parts and adds a brief poetic description of form or function of each. In the process it reveals particular insights which place it after the work of Herophilus and Erasistratus. The useless spleen,[89] the bladder woven from vessels,[90] are suggestive, as also, perhaps the notion that swallowing is accomplished by a shove rather than attraction.[91] The claim that the brain, in its acropolis, gives directions to the limbs through the nerves, places it definitively after the Alexandrian anatomists' discovery of the nervous system. The advanced anatomy is used casually, not in self-conscious display that it is modern. Nor is there emphasis on teleology and the wisdom of the artificer, as in Plato, Aristotle and Galen. It is a modest, reverent appreciation of the organs that serve us and an appreciation of the terminology.

Letter 24 promises to do, but does not do, what is done by surviving works on dietetics, of which our best examples are the Hippocratic *Regimen* and Galen's *Hygiene*. The Letter of Diocles to King Antigonus which is offered by Paulus Aegineta 1.99, is a brief, summary version of a regimen. In its effect, Letter 24 reads like a cover letter for a regimen, containing a few relevant general principles that are introductory to such a work. The provenience of the general principles is not obvious. The division of diseases into the types *kata genos* and *kata pathos* has no direct parallel, and the purpose of the division is not clear. The principle that desires for nutriment and also diseases come from opposites is good doctrine from the Hippocratic Corpus. The writer draws from the Corpus his illustrations for the principle that diseases resolve diseases, but his terminology for the principle, expressed in Ilberg's excellent emendation, νούσους ὑπὸ νούσων λυομένας, is not directly paralleled elsewhere.

Attempts to place this letter have not been notably successful. Herman De Ley concludes that the addressee is Demetrius Poliorketes, father of Antigonus Gonatas.[92] In this he follows Felix Heinimann, who says that this letter and the letter from Diocles to Antigonus preserved by Paulus Aegineta are of the same

---

[88] Celsus, *De medicina*, Proem. 7-10, Erotian, *Vocum Hippocraticarum Collectio*, ed., Ernst Nachmanson (Göteborg: 1918) p. 3, ὅσοιγε λογικῆς ἀντιποιοῦνται. The similarity to the expression in the letter seems noteworthy, and I do not find a similar phrase elsewhere.

[89] Erasistratus seems to have said that the spleen is good for nothing (ἐγένετο μάτην): Galen, *Usefulness of the Parts* 3.315 K. and *Natural Faculties* 2.91 K.

[90] Erasistratus said that the compound organs were woven from veins, arteries, and sinews, with nutriment poured into the container thus formed (παρέγχυμα). Cf. Galen, *Nat. Fac.* 2.96 K., *Anonymus Londinensis* chapt XXI, Pseudo-Galen *Introductio sive medicus* 14.697-8 K., Soranus, *Gyn.* 3.4.

[91] Cf. Galen, *Nat. Fac.* 2.60 K.

[92] De Ley, pp. 73-76.

period, possibly by the same author.[93] De Ley associates this letter with 23, the anatomy, and hence would date both to the last quarter of the fourth century B.C. As we have seen above, that dating is far too early for the anatomy. Because the author of 24, (which claims to be a letter from Hippocrates) claims authorship of 23 (which claims to be from Democritus), other conjectures about the change in attribution are also required. I think that we need not take very seriously the possibility of a relationship of date and/or author between the Hippocratic Letter to Demetrius and the 'Diocles' letter to Antigonus. The names of the addressees are the closest link between the two letters. Both address the subject of staying free from disease, the theory of which is laid out in the Hippocratic *Regimen*. But the Hippocratic letter is only an exercise in the proem to such a letter, while the 'Diocles' letter has its own proem and the prescriptions that it implies. The 'Diocles' letter describes the symptoms that appear on the development of an affection in any of the four regions, head, chest, intestines or urinary system, and gives prescriptions, mostly purges, intended to avert serious illness. And it also gives a general regimen for the year according to hot, cold, wet, and dry aspects of the seasons, the year being divided into six parts. Another extant letter, entitled Hippocrates or Diocles to king Ptolemy, gives much the same material in a different order with some verbal differences, and that may shed light on the history of the 'Diocles' letter, but none, I think, on the Hippocratic Letter 24.[94] The letters differ in style enough that we need not assert that the Hippocratic letter is an introduction to the 'Diocles' letter, nor that the 'Diocles' letter is an expanded version of the Hippocratic one.

---

[93] Felix Heinimann, "Diokles von Karystos und der prophylaktische Brief an König Antigonos", *Museum Helveticum* 12 (1955) 158-172. The Diocles letter was edited by Werner Jaeger, *Diokles von Karystos* (Berlin: 1938) pp. 75-78. Heinimann argues against Jaeger's acceptance of the Diocles letter as genuine and denies that the addressee is Antigonus Monophthalmus. Rather, he says, the philosophic qualities attributed to the addressee seem to fit Gonatas, as Arnaldo Momigliano argued, "Una lettera a Claudio e una lettera ad Antigona Gonata", *Athenaeum* 11 (1933) 132-135. But Heinimann rejects Momigliano's notion (which follows Wellmann) that the author is Aristogenes.

[94] Published in J. F. Boissonade, *Anecdota Graeca III* (Paris 1831) 422-428. A scribe at some point in the tradition of ms. b wrote after letter 24, "We should look for the rest of this letter and the whole of the one to Ptolemy". This observation seems perceptive on two counts: he read 24 as a cover letter, and he was aware of the other dietetic letter. It does not prove anything about the ultimate origin of the letters, though it could possibly say something about the formation of the collection that ms. b offers.

THE TEXT AND THE MANUSCRIPTS

The peculiar history of these writings is reflected in their odd textual history. There was never a complete collection of the Hippocratic pseudepigrapha before the publication of the Aldine edition of Hippocrates. Two distinct textual traditions descend from antiquity: the manuscripts that carry the medical writings of the Corpus Hippocraticum carry the Epibomios and Presbeutikos and the Athenian Decree, numbers 25-27, preceded by letters 1-22; manuscripts of the epistolographic tradition, which carry various collections of letters, all lack the two speeches, and exhibit several different selections of letters: Pal. gr. 398, the oldest by five centuries,[95] contains 1-24, and also 25, which it has between 9 and 10. The next oldest, Vat. gr. 1300, of the fourteenth century, has only 1-5 and 11-17, a collection characteristic of a number of Renaissance manuscripts.[96] The papyri of the second century A.D. also lack 6-10, which might make us suspect that this is an old selection. Vat. gr. 1354, of the fifteenth century, in company with other Renaissance manuscripts, has 1-5, 11-18, 20 and 22.[97] Parisinus gr. 3052, of the sixteenth century, has 3-9. Its omission of 1-2 is reminiscent of the papyri, with which, as I am about to say, it has affinities also in its text of letters 4 and 5.

Alternative versions of letters 4 and 5, already apparent in the papyri, further complicate the manuscript groupings. In the pair I designate 4 and 5 Hystanes says that he is forwarding the king's letter, and Hippocrates writes in response to "the letter you said came from the king." In the pair I designate 4a and 5a there is no mention of the king's letter: Hystanes says that the king desires Hippocrates to come, and Hippocrates tells him to tell the king "No." The pairs 4 and 5 or 4a and 5a should logically appear together, but the groups of manuscripts ring all possible changes:

Papyrus 1:	4 and 5
Papyri 2 and 3, and Par. gr. 3052:	4a and 5a
Mss. of the medical trad., MUV and Pal. gr. 398 (b):	4 and 5a
Other mss. of the epistolographic tradition besides b:	4a and 5

In addition, papyrus 1 has 4a in its margin and papyrus 2 has 5 in its text following 5a.

Though the complexities of the manuscript tradition go back to antiquity, it is not immediately obvious how the divisions between manuscript groups

---

[95] Ms. Pal. gr. 398 was copied in Constaninople in the mid-ninth century. See N. G. Wilson, *Scholars of Byzantium* (Oxford: 1983) 87-8.

[96] Other manuscripts of this group are Laur. Plut. 59.27, Mutinensis 54 (III B 2), Parisinus 2652 (Littré's ο), Parisinus 3050 (Littré's υ). [See note 101 below.]

[97] This group is exhibited by the following fifteenth and sixteenth century mss.: Bononensis 3563, Conv. Sopp. 153, Laur. Plut. 57.12, 57.45, and 59.5, Mutinensis 191, and Parisini 2755 (Littré's σ), 3047 (Littré's τ), 1760 (Littré's ω), and Paris.205 Sup. (Littré's ψ).

developed. We are not seeing a case in which a brief selection was made out of a larger corpus, but perhaps rather a result of the piecemeal growth of the collection.

MANUSCRIPT EVIDENCE

Manuscripts of the Medical Tradition

Three of the independent ancient Hippocratic manuscripts have the pseudepigrapha, one lacks them entirely, and one has only the *Speech from the Altar*.

Designation		Date	Contents
M	Marcianus graecus 269[98]	saec. X	1-3, 4, 5a, 6-22, 25-27
Θ	Vindobonensis Med. gr. 4	saec. X-XI[99]	no pseudepigrapha
A	Parisinus graecus 2253	saec. XI	26
U	Urbinas graecus 64[100]	saec. XII	1-3, 4, 5a, 6-22, 25-27
V	Vaticanus graecus 276	saec. XII	1-3, 4, 5a, 6-22, 25-27

---

[98] M is mutilated at the end, and has lost most of the text of the *Presbeutikos*. Where M is defective, I use three mss. of the M tradition in its stead:

I	Parisinus graecus 2140	saec. XIII	1-3, 4, 5a, 6-19 init., 26-27
H^b	Parisinus graecus 2142	saec. XIV	1-3, 4, 5a, 6-18, 26-27, 25, 19, 20, 21, 23, 22
G	Parisinus graecus 2141	saec. XIV	1-3, 4, 5a, 6-19 init., 26-27

Ms. I, a copy of M, is the source of H^b (i.e., the second and later part of H) and of G. In its original form it apparently had the full text of M, including the end of 27, but it lost some folios before they were copied. See Jacques Jouanna, "L' Analyse codicologique du Parisinus gr. 2140 et l' histoire du texte hippocratique," *Scriptorium* 38 (1984) 50-67. H^b appears to have copied the penultimate page of I before its loss (Jouanna p. 58-9); G lacked two folios of I, and restored them from elsewhere (one does not know whence). H^b filled the gap left by I's loss of earlier folios by copying 19-23 and 25 from a ms. of the b tradition, but not from b itself. I use the text of H to supplement the evidence of b and c in 23.

[99] N. G. Wilson, *Scholars of Byzantium*, p. 148, places this book in the reign of Basil II in Constantinople.

[100] This ms. was designated X by J. Heiberg in *Hippocrates*, CMG I 1 (Leipzig and Berlin: 1927), Vat. by J. Jouanna, *Hippocrate, Des Vents. De l'Art*, Budé V.1 (Paris: 1988). For descriptions and dating see Jouanna, p. 52, and B. Alexanderson, *Die Hippokratische Schrift Prognostikon* (Göteborg: 1963) 87. It is a Greek-Italian manuscript from the area of Reggio, N.G. Wilson, *Scholars of Byzantium*, p. 212.

Manuscripts of the Epistolographic Tradition

No definitive study of these manuscripts has been done, and I do not have a complete inventory.[101] I have chosen the best representatives of the groups that I found.

Designation		Date	Contents
b	Palatinus graecus 398	saec. IX	1-3, 4, 5a, 6-9, 25, 10-24
a	Vaticanus graecus 1309	saec. XIV	1-3, 4a, 5, 11-17
c	Vaticanus graecus 1353	saec. XV	1-3, 4a, 5, 6-9, 11-18, 20, 22 (+ marg. 25, 10, 19, 21, 23-24)
d	Vaticanus graecus 1354	saec. XV	1-3, 4a, 5, 11-18, 20, 22, 6-10
φ	Parisinus graecus 3052	saec. XVI	3-9

Papyri

p^1	P. Oxy. IX 1184v	s. I A.D.	3, 4, 5, 6a (and in marg. 4a)
p^2	P. Berol. Inv. 7094v	s. II-III A.D.	3, 4a, 5a, 5, 11
p^3	P. Berol. Inv. 21137v P. Berol. Inv. 6934v	s. II-III A.D.	3, 4a, 5a, 5, 11

Manuscripts of the Medical Tradition

The oldest and best manuscripts which contain the works of the Hippocratic Corpus, as well as other medical writings, are AMUV. Ms. A contains, from the Pseudepigrapha, only 26, the *Speech at the Altar*. The others contain all the Pseudepigrapha save for 23 and 24. H, a recentior of the M tradition, has 23, in a text not copied directly from either of the other two extant sources, b and c. Ms. M is mutilated towards the end, in 27. For the tradition of M, where M is missing, I use GHI, recentiores of the M tradition.[102] Of these three, first I,

---

[101] While this book was in the press, there appeared D. Th. Sakalis, ΙΠΠΟΚΡΑΤΟΥΣ ΕΠΙΣΤΟΛΑΙ, ῾Εκδοση κριτική και ερμηνευτική, Ioannina, 1989, which includes an extensive account, with a proposed stemma codicum, of the manuscripts which contain the Hippocratic Letters (1-24). His information should be added to what I give here.

My manuscripts acd = O represent Sakalis' epistolographic E family, while my ms. φ comes from his other epistolographic family, ε.

[102] For descriptions of MIVH, see *Ippocrate, Epidemie Libro Sesto*, a cura di Daniela Manetti e Amneris Roselli (Florence, 1982, *Biblioteca di Studi Superiori* LXVI) xxv-xxxviii. Cay Lienau, ed., *Hippocratis De Superfetatione*, *CMG* I.2.2 (Berlin 1973) distinguishes older and younger parts of manuscript V, to the younger part of which (V^b) the Pseudepigrapha belong, and similarly older and younger parts of H are distinguished by Hermann Grensemann as H^a and H^b, *Über Achtmonatskinder, Über das Siebenmonatskind (unecht)* CMG I 2, 1 (Berlin: 1968). For a study of the relations of the recentiores to M, and the scribal corrections and conjectures that they exhibit, see J. Irigoin, "Le rôle des recentiores dans l' établissement du texte hippocratique," *Corpus Hippocraticum, Colloque de Mons*, ed. R. Joly (Mons 1977) 9-17, and S. Byl, "Les

then H fails, leaving G as the only representative of the M tradition at the end. (I do not cite GHI when M is available.)

Manuscripts of the Epistolographic Tradition

All the Pseudepigrapha, save for 26 and 27 (*Speech at the Altar*, and *Embassy*) come to us also in manuscripts of the epistolographic tradition, which, besides Hippocratic Letters, contain collections of letters attributed to well known figures of antiquity, Euripides, Heraclitus, Diogenes, etc. The two lines of transmission for the Hippocratic letters existed separately from at least the first century A.D. The epistolographic tradition for Hippocratic letters itself seems to have been split early into several branches which contained different selections of letters, the fullest represented by ms. b, which uniquely contains 23 and 24, the next fullest by my manuscripts c and d, and the next by the tradition that provides the majority of our Renaissance epistolographic mss., as in my ms. a, and the smallest by ms. φ.[103] For the epistolographic tradition, Littré used , in addition to b and φ, seven fifteenth and sixteenth century Paris manuscripts which he designated οστυχψω. Putzger used the same epistolographic manuscripts as Littré, which Littré reported accurately.[104] My mss. acd, along with b, are intended to represent the available tradition in the epistolographic manuscripts. a is of the same type as Littré's οστυχψω, carrying the same letters and essentially the same text, and it is older than they, though I have not been able to establish that any of them were copied directly from it. Mss. c and d are of a type that is not represented among the Paris mss., an expanded collection that adds letters 18, 20, and 22 to those of a. c is additionally of interest because it has a marginal addition which is like the text of b, but independent of it, and therefore can broaden our evidence of those treatises for which b has been the only witness. Littré's ms. φ, which uniquely of the epistolographic group contains the selection letters 3-9, is erratic in its text, but has seemed to be worth reporting because it

---

recentiores du traité pseudo-hippocratique Du *Régime*; quelques problèmes," *Hippocratica, Actes du Colloque Hippocratique de Paris*, ed. M. Grmek (Paris 1980) 73-83. Manuscript U is described by Putzger, p. V. Manuscript G was used by Asulanus for the Aldine edition of Hippocrates (note the apparatus for p. 110, line 20, 122.2, etc.). It has a number of conjectures and proposed corrections. Jacques Jouanna, *Scriptorium* 38 (1984) 56-9, establishes that H^b and G were copied from ms. I after it had lost a number of folios.

[103] Manuscript b is described by Putzger on p. V of his edition, and in H. Stevenson, *Codices manuscripti Palatini Graeci Bibliothecae Vaticanae* (Rome 1885) 254-57. Descriptions of a, c, and d are given by Ingemar Düring, *Chion of Heraclea* pp. 29-30, and good physical descriptions of the manuscripts by Sabatucci, 380-391. For their affiliation, see, e.g., apparatus to page 78 line 23 below: post ὅκως add. ἢ abcd, om. MUV, and in the same line λεχθέντα MUVb, λαληθέντα acd, and p. 62, line 12: τε MUV δὲ acd om. b. In d the text of letters 6-10, readings from which I report, was added after letter 22 by the same hand as the preceding, but apparently from a different source. d's text in these added letters is closer to the text of the medical than the epistolographic tradition.

[104] Putzger appears to have codified Littré's information by using r and R for many and all of οστυχψω. He states wrongly (p.VI) that they contain Letter 10.

has affinities with the papyri. The statement that it contains unique memory of true readings, however, has seemed to me optimistic.[105] The papyrus texts of the Letters represent different early selections of letters from the epistolographic tradition.[106] The text they carry is related to both the medical and epistolographic tradition, which one can infer is a sign that they come early in the divided tradition.

We can best approach the history of the whole collection through its parts. We start from the likelihood that there was never a full collection of letters, speeches and decrees from which selections were made, but groups that were assembled at various times into different collections. The nature of the groups can perhaps shed light on the order of composition of the letters, if not the absolute dates.

25-27

As I argued above, the speeches, 27 and 26, are the oldest pseudepigrapha, and were part of the Hippocratic collection in the Alexandrian Library. 25, the Athenian Decree, was added at some point to illustrate them. Why, one asks, does A have only 26, and not 25-27 like the other medical manuscripts, MUV, or like Θ, none at all? And why is b alone of the epistolographic group in having 25, and if it has 25, why not 26 and 27? Such quizzical questions sometimes admit of convincing answers, sometimes do not. In the case of 25-27, it seems reasonable that the copyist of Θ, or of an ancestor, creating a practical medical manuscript, passed the pseudepigrapha by entirely, and the scribe of A, or its ancestor, who was writing Hippocratic material, took the speech of Hippocrates, but rejected that of Thessalos and the decree, while the branch represented by MUV, interested in biography as well as medical works, kept all three. Some scribe of an ancestor of b, a systematic collector of letters relating to Hippocrates, copied 25, the decree, and placed it in the most reasonable place for it in b's collection, after the Persian letters, because it refers to Hippocrates' rejection of Persian overtures, and it offers similarities and contrasts with 9, the Coan decree, which it follows in b's collection. But 26 and 27, being speeches, were rejected as inappropriate to an epistolographic collection. c is a manuscript of the type of a, but after it was copied it was augmented in the margin with letters from the b collection, in the order of b, 25, 10, 19, 21, 23 and 24. The text of these supplements in c shows that they were not copied into c from b itself, though b is three centuries older than c, but from a relative. Thus we can speak of a b tradition.

---

[105] φ agrees with now one, now another of the papyri in its readings, see, e.g., apparatus, p. 50, lines 16, 19, 62.6,7,8, etc.

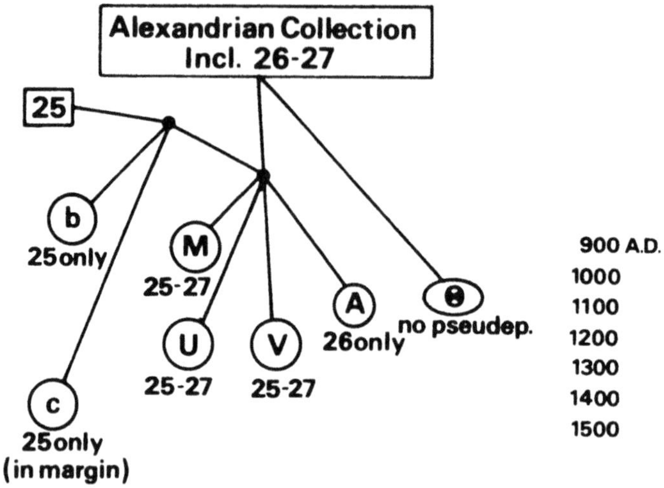

10-21

The Democritus sequence, as one infers from the occurrences of the letters in the manuscripts, divides into the basic group 11-17, and additions, 10 and 18-21, of which 10, 18, and 20 are letters, and 19 and 21 are the discourses on madness and hellebore. 10 is the letter from the Abderites that 11 from Hippocrates answers, and it is of comparable quality with 11-17, but its weak representation in the epistolographic tradition sets it apart. It is clearly missing from the papyrus collections, which have 3-5 and 11, and they might or might not have had others beyond 11. It seems possible, though not likely, that out of an original, complete collection, a selection of "Hippocratic Letters" would reject 10. I am therefore inclined to conclude that 10 is a later addition to 11-17. The treatises 19 and 21 are pastiches, and 18 and 20 are cover letters for them. Do we infer from their manuscript occurrences that 21 is the last written, and thus probably 19 also was written after 18 and 20,and that the whole sequence 18-21 is an exchange between Democritus and Hippocrates which is inferior to, and written later than, 11-17? b has the whole group, 10-21, d lacks 10 and 19, c lacks 10, 19 and 21, and a lacks 10 and 18-21. b and the medical tradition have them all. 22, the letter to Thessalos, appears wherever 20 does.

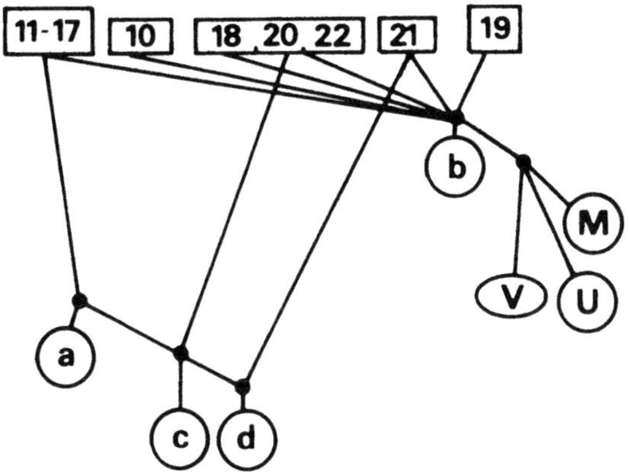

1-9

The Persian Letters offer the most complex pattern in the manuscript selection, even more interesting because the complexities show up early, and are even greater in the papyrus manuscripts which come near the beginning of the tradition. Letters 4 and 5 appear in two versions. The pair that I designate 4 and 5 relate to the forwarding of the king's letter to Hippocrates and his answering it as "the letter you said came from the king." 4a and 5a do not refer to a letter from the king. Instead, Hystanes conveys to Hippocrates the king's desire for him, and Hippocrates replies with a summary dismissal. The various groups of manuscripts have different choices from these two pairs of letters, but they do not choose only the logical pairs. The papyrus mss. have logical pairs, and p^1, which has 4 and 5, has 4a also in its margin, while p^2 has 4a and 5a and 5 in that order. On the other hand the mss. of the medical tradition have 4 and 5a, while the epistolographic group represented by acd have 4a and 5. Ms. b, the most venerable of the epistolographic mss. has 4 and 5a, unlike the bulk of the epistolographic mss., and like those of the medical tradition, and φ, a late epistolographic ms. has 4a and 5a, like the papyri p^2 and p^3. Letters 6-9 do not appear in the papyri or in a and d, but they are in c, and also in b and the medical tradition. And they are in φ. φ, like all three of the papyri, lacks 1 and 2, while the other mss. of the epistolographic and medical traditions have them. The rationale is not obvious.

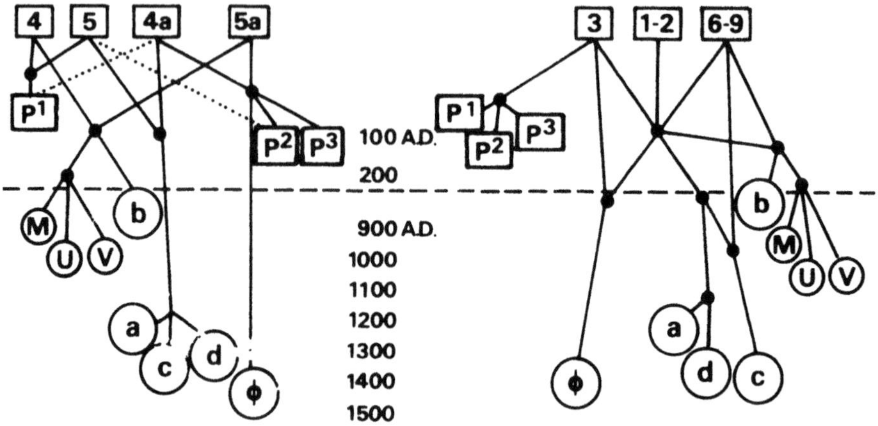

23-24

Finally, 23 and 24 appear only in b and in c's marginal addition, and 23 appears in H, a manuscript of the medical tradition which is derived from M or a close relative of M, but is eclectic in its text in the pseudepigrapha.[107] H's text of 23 and c's text of 23 and 24 are not taken directly from b. They are independently derived from a relative or relatives of b. H could have taken its text of 23, the fanciful anatomy attributed to Democritus, from a source that had both 23 and 24, while rejecting 24, the hygiene to Demetrius attributed to Hippocrates, but a reason for doing so is not apparent, and one is at liberty to conclude that H's source lacked 24. The order of H's texts of the pseudepigrapha suggests a search for a complete collection.[108]

---

[107] H has the M text of 26 and 27, but in the rest has a contaminated text similar to b and to c.

[108] H's order for the pseudepigrapha is 1-18 (fol. 530-540), 26-27 (fol. 540-543v), 544 blank, and, in another hand, 25, 19, 20, 21, 23, 22 (fol. 544v-546v).

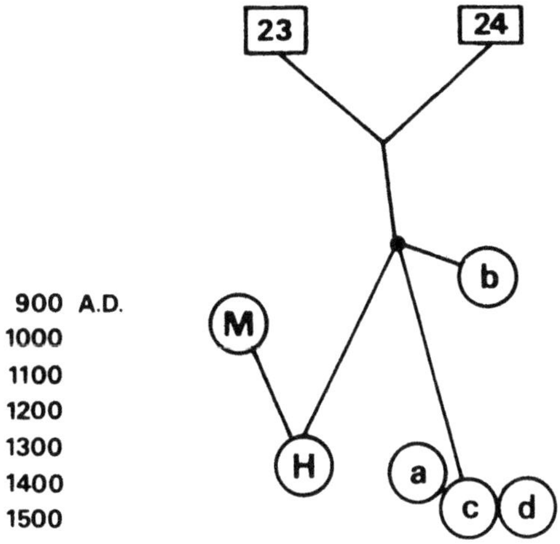

I have not found it possible to combine all these elements into a single graph or stemma to show relationships. Indeed, I cannot say what the history is that a stemma should clarify.

Secondary Tradition

The secondary tradition for the text of the pseudepigrapha is very thin. Erotian cites ten words from the *Presbeutikos*, identified by Ernst Nachmanson, *Erotianstudien*, Uppsala: Almquist & Wiksell, 1917, pp. 440-441. There are a number of indirect references to the contents of the letters, but little evidence for the text.

Dialect

The Ionic Dialect of the Hippocratic Corpus is not a spoken language, but a book language whose original forms cannot be known because of successive corruptions and corrections of the words in the process of the transmission of the texts. All the sources of the text, including the earliest papyrus manuscripts, exhibit considerable inconsistency in their use of the Dialect. This is even more true for the *Pseudepigrapha* than it is for the medical works. It is likely that the dialect was, to some degree, mixed in the original writings, and that the Ionic, as an affectation, was a matter of flavor about which the authors and the later scribes were more self-conscious at some times, and with some words than others.[109] The process of adjusting the dialect seems to have been repeated in each generation as the texts were copied, and recovery of the original has been put beyond our reach.[110] A scholarly consensus, with which I am in accord, has developed whereby, in addition to following the tendencies of the best manuscript or manuscripts, editors introduce corrections for a general consistency of inflectional form, αὐτοῖσι, not αὐτοῖς, ποιέουσι, not ποιοῦσι, etc., and remove the clear hyper-Ionisms, those erroneous forms that have apparently been introduced into the text by scribes as elegant "corrections". I have admitted some inconsistency into my text. I have only rarely reported manuscript variations in orthography, when they seemed interesting or where they might be preferable to the text I print.

Enclitics

For accentuation of enclitics I have followed the principles enunciated by W. S. Barrett, *Euripides Hippolytus* (Oxford,1964) 424-427. In the few cases in which enclitics come in series I treat the group as an accentual unit, e.g., ἦγόν τε με.

---

109 There were discussions of, and disagreements about, the dialect in the ancient commentators and editors, about which we get some, but not much, information from Galen. See his commentary on *Fractures* 18B 322 Kühn, in which he says that some commentators treated the dialect as Old Attic, and his commentary on *Epidemics 6*, CMG 5.10.2.2, p. 483, where he tells us that the editors Dioscurides and Capiton presented all Hippocrates' works in the Coan dialect (as they understood it). We cannot attain the truth or locate the Ionic dialect in such cases as p. 62, line 9, in letter 12: ἀπανθρωπεῦνται V ἀπανθρωπέονται U ἀπανθρωποῦνται b ἀπανθρωπεύονται acd.

Ms. b has many suggestions written into it, some apparently from other manuscripts and some original with the corrector himself. I cite only the most interesting.

110 See the discussions of medical Ionic by Hugo Kühlewein, *Hippocratis opera quae feruntur omnia*, vol. 1 (Leipzig: Teubner, 1894), pp. LXV-CCXXVIII, E. Schwyzer in Karl Deichgräber, ed., *Hippocratis de carnibus* (Leipzig and Berlin: 1935) 62-70, Hans Diller, ed., *Hippocratis De aere aquis locis*, CMG 1.1.2 (Berlin: 1970) 13-17, and Jacques Jouanna, ed., *Hippocratis De natura hominis*, CMG 1.1.3 (Berlin: 1975) 133-155.

EDITIONS

Letters 1-5, 11-18 and 20 were first edited by M. Musurus and printed by Aldus Manutius in 1499 in a volume of ancient letters: *Epistolae diversorum philosophorum*. The first collected Latin translation of *Hippocrates* by Fabius Calvus, Rome: 1525, contains 1-22, 25-27. The Aldine Greek princeps of Hippocrates, edited by F. Asulanus, Venice: 1526, exhibits the complete series, 1-27, for the first time. All subsequent editors of the corpus include the pseudepigrapha in this form and sequence. The most important of these are:

Asul.	*Omnia opera Hippocratis*, Venetiis in aedibus Aldi et Andreae Asulani, 1526
Corn.	*Hippocratis Coi libri omnes*, Froben, Basileae, 1538 (edited by Janus Cornarius)
Merc.	*Hippocratis Coi opera quae existunt*, ed. Hieronymus Mercurialis, Venetiis, 1588
Foës	*Magni Hippocratis opera omnia quae exstant*, ed. Anutius Foesius. Francofurti, 1595
Lind.	*Magni Hippocratis Coi opera omnia Graece et Latine*, ed., Ioan. Anton. van der Linden, Leiden: 1665
Li.	*Oeuvres complètes d'Hippocrate* par Émile Littré, vol. 9, Paris:1861.
Ermerins	*Hippocratis et aliorum medicorum veterum reliquiae*, ed. Franciscus Z. Ermerins, Traiecti ad Rhen. 1859-64.
Hercher	*Epistolographi Graeci*, recens. R. Hercher, Parisiis 1878.
Putz.	Walter Putzger, *Hippocratis quae feruntur epistulae ad codicum fidem recensitae*, Programm Wurzen, Leipzig: Teubner, 1914

Foës used a number of manuscripts and much medical insight and philological ingenuity to improve the text of the early editions, which were based on manuscripts of the M tradition. Littré extended the manuscript evidence greatly with the manuscripts in Paris, including his C (Parisinus 2146), which is a copy of V, eight Paris manuscripts of the epistolographic tradition, and a (less than perfect) collation of b (Palatinus 398) made for him by a Prof. Roullez of Brussels. Putzger, whose edition contains only 1-25, added also U.[111] Editions between Foës and Littré used Foës's reports of readings and his copious notes, and similarly Ermerins and Hercher depended on the full apparatus of Littré for their information about the tradition of the text, as Putzger may have for his report of the Paris epistolographic manuscripts, for whose evidence he cared little.

[111] Through the kindness of Fridolf Kudlien and Jutta Harig-Kollesch I have been able to see Putzger's preliminary text for 26 and 27, which is stored at the Akademie der Wissenschaften in Berlin.

SIGLA

p^1	P. Oxy. IX 1184v	s. I A.D.
p^2	P. Berol. Inv. 7094v	s. II/III A.D.
p^3	P. Berol. Inv. 21137v and 6934v	s. II/III A.D.
b	Palatinus graecus 398	saec. IX
M	Marcianus graecus 269	saec. X
A	Parisinus graecus 2253	saec. XI
U	Urbinas graecus 64	saec. XII
V	Vaticanus graecus 276	saec. XII
I	Parisinus graecus 2140	saec. XIII
G	Parisinus graecus 2141	saec. XIV
H	Parisinus graecus 2142	saec. XIV
a	Vaticanus graecus 1309	saec. XIV
c	Vaticanus graecus 1353	saec. XV
d	Vaticanus graecus 1354	saec. XV
O	= agreement of acd	
φ	Parisinus graecus 3052	saec. XVI
Diels	H. Diels, Fragmente der Vorsokratiker ^{6}, Berlin: 1951	
Erot.	Erotian, ed. Ernst Nachmanson, Uppsala: 1918	
Paton	W. R. Paton, in , W. R. Paton and E. L. Hicks, *The Inscriptions of Cos*, Oxford: 1891.	

I am the first to make use of manuscripts a, c, and d for the Hippocratic text, and to employ those symbols for them. b, the oldest and best in its class would normally be designated a, but I have retained Littré's siglum for it, as I have also for φ.

ΤΟΥ ΙΠΠΟΚΡΑΤΟΥΣ

ΕΠΙΣΤΟΛΑΙ ΠΡΕΣΒΕΥΤΙΚΟΣ ΕΠΙΒΩΜΙΟΣ ΔΟΓΜΑ

ΕΠΙΣΤΟΛΑΙ ΠΡΕΣΒΕΥΤΙΚΟΣ ΕΠΙΒΩΜΙΟΣ ΔΟΓΜΑ

Littré IX 1. Βασιλεὺς βασιλέων μέγας Ἀρταξέρξης Παίτῳ χαίρειν·

312 Νοῦσος προσεπέλασεν ἡ καλουμένη λοιμικὴ τοῖς στρατεύμασιν ἡμῶν καὶ πολλὰ ποιησάντων ἡμῶν ἔνδοσιν οὐκ ἔδωκεν. ὅθεν ἀξιῶ παντοίως καὶ πάσαις ταῖς παρ' ἐμοῦ διδομέναις δωρεαῖς, ἤτοι τῶν ἐκ φύσεώς σου ἐπινοήμασιν ἤτοι τῶν ἐκ τέχνης πρήξεων ἤτοι ἑτέρου ἀνδρὸς ἑρμηνείην δυναμένου ἰήσασθαι πέμπε τάχος. μάστιξον, ἀξιῶ, τὸ πάθος. ἀλύκη γὰρ κατὰ τῶν ὄχλων καὶ πολὺς ἅλυς πνεῦμα μέγα καὶ πυκνὸν ἔχων. οὐ πολεμοῦντες πολεμούμεθα, ἐχθρὸν ἔχοντες τὸν θῆρα λυμαινόμενον τὰ ποίμνια. τέτρωκε πολλούς, δυσιάτους ἐποίησε· πικρὰ βέλη βελῶν καταπέμπει. οὐ φέρω. γνώμην οὐκέτι ἔχω μετ' ἀνδρῶν γονίμων βουλεύσασθαι. λῦε ταῦτα πάντα μὴ διαλείψας ἀγαθῇ συνειδήσει. ἔρρωσο.

2. Παῖτος βασιλεῖ μεγάλῳ Ἀρταξέρξῃ χαίρειν·

Τὰ φυσικὰ βοηθήματα οὐ λύει τὴν ἐπιδημίαν λοιμικοῦ πάθους. ἃ δὲ ἐκ φύσεως γίνεται νοσήματα, αὐτὴ ἡ φύσις ἴηται κρίνουσα· ὅσα δὲ ἐξ ἐπιδημίης, τέχνη τεχνικῶς κρίνουσα τὴν τροπὴν τῶν σωμάτων.
314 Ἱπποκράτης δὲ ἰητρὸς ἴῆται τοῦτο τὸ πάθος. τῷ γένει μὲν | οὖν ἐστι Δωριεύς, πόλεως δὲ Κῶ, πατρὸς δὲ Ἡρακλείδα τοῦ Ἱπποκράτους τοῦ Γνωσιδίκου τοῦ Νέβρου τοῦ Σωστράτου τοῦ Θεοδώρου τοῦ Κλεομυττάδα τοῦ Κρισάμιδος. οὗτος θείᾳ φύσει κέχρηται καὶ ἐκ μικρῶν καὶ ἰδιωτικῶν εἰς μεγάλα καὶ τεχνικὰ προήγαγε τὴν ἰητρικήν. γίνεται μὲν οὖν ὁ θεῖος Ἱπποκράτης ἔνατος μὲν ἀπὸ Κρισάμιδος τοῦ βασιλέως, ὀκτωκαιδέκατος δὲ ἀπὸ Ἀσκληπιοῦ, εἰκοστὸς δὲ ἀπὸ Διός, μητρὸς δὲ Πραξιθέας τῆς Φαιναρέτης ἐκ τῆς οἰκίας τῶν Ἡρακλειδῶν, ὥστε κατὰ ἀμφότερα τὰ σπέρματα θεῶν ἀπόγονός ἐστιν ὁ θεῖος Ἱπποκράτης, πρὸς μὲν πατρὸς Ἀσκληπιάδης ὤν, πρὸς δὲ μητρὸς Ἡρακλείδης. ἔμαθε δὲ τὴν τέχνην παρά τε τῷ πατρὶ Ἡρακλείδῃ καὶ παρὰ τῷ πάππῳ Ἱπποκράτει. ἀλλὰ παρὰ μὲν τούτοις, ὡς εἰκός, τὰ πρῶτα ἐμυήθη τῆς ἰητρικῆς, ὅσα πιθανὸν ἦν καὶ τούτους εἰδέναι. τὴν δὲ σύμπασαν τέχνην αὐτὸς ἑωυτὸν ἐδιδάξατο

Epistulae 1-2. Mss. MUVbO (O = acd) 1 πέτω MVb || 3 post πολλὰ add. πολλάκις bO || 4 σου om. O || 5 ἐπινοημάτων UbO ante τέχης add. τῆς V || 6 ταχέως U μαστίζον M μαστίζειν U ἅλωκε MVO ἅλωκεν b ἅλωκα U corr. Li. || 7 τὸν ὄχλον UO πολλὸς ἁλὺς b || 8-9 τὸ ποίμνιον V || 11: λύε bO λύεται MV λύε τὲ U corr. Li. συνειδήσει: τύχη O || 13 post βασιλεῖ add. βασιλέων τῷ MUVb post μεγάλῳ add. δεσπότῃ MUVb || 14 in marg. γρ. νοσήματα λύσει b τοῦ λοιμ. bO ἃ δὲ: ὅσα δὲ b ὅσα γὰρ O || 16 ante τῶν add τὴν. b || 18 πατρὸς: ἰητρὸς MUV Ἡρακλείδου O || 21 post οὖν add. ἡμῖν bO || 23 τοῦ Ἀσκ. O || 25 θεαπόγονός b 26 ἔμαθέ τε bO || 27 τε om. ac ἡρακλείδᾳ bO Ἱπποκράτη U || 28 τούτων b (corr. b^2) ὃς ἀπίθανον MUV ὅσα πιθανὰ b || 29 ἐδίδαξεν Ob (corr b^2)

LETTERS, EMBASSY, SPEECH FROM THE ALTAR, DECREE

1. King of Kings, great Artaxerxes to Paitus. Greetings

The disease called plague has descended on our army. Though we have done much, it has given no relief. Therefore, I ask, in all ways and by all the gifts given by me, send me something quickly: natural remedies from your own knowledge, some procedure of science, or an explanation by some other man who can cure it. Scourge the affection, I beg. Breathing heavily, anguish and despair have invaded the multitude. We are beaten without striking a blow. Our enemy is a beast ravaging our flocks. It has wounded many, put them beyond healing. It sends down dart after bitter dart. I cannot bear it. I no longer have the mind to take counsel with men of quality. Stop all this, omitting nothing, with your good understanding. Be well!

2. Paitus to the great king Artaxerxes. Greetings.

Natural remedies do not get rid of the visitation of the plague epidemic. Diseases from nature, nature herself judges (brings to a crisis) and heals. Those from a visitation the science heals, judging scientifically the alterations of bodies. Hippocrates the physician cures this malady. By family he is Dorian, of the city Cos, son of Heraclides, son of Gnosidicus, son of Nebros, son of Sostratus, son of Theodorus, son of Cleomyttades, son of Crisamis. He has a divine nature, and he has brought forth the healing science from minor, idiosyncratic activities to great scientific ones.[1]/The divine Hippocrates is eighth, you know, from King Crisamis, seventeenth from Asclepius, nineteenth from Zeus, and his mother is Phainarete's daughter Praxithea, from the Heraclid house.[2]

Hence, by the seed of both sides, the divine Hippocrates is descended from gods, from Asclepius by his father, from Heracles by his mother. He learned the science from his father Heraclides and from his grandfather Hippocrates. It seems likely that he was first initiated by them into the first mysteries of the science, which it is credible that even they knew, but he taught the total science to

---

[1] With the phrase ἐκ μικρῶν καὶ ἰδιωτικῶν εἰς μεγάλα καὶ τεχνικὰ προήγαγε it is possible that the author suggests that Hippocrates brought others outside the family into the profession, as Galen suggests in *Anatomical Procedures* (*Anat. Admin.*, Kühn 2.280-281), but more likely he means simply what is developed below, that he somehow reconstituted and objectified medical theory, which had before been peculiar to each practitioner.

[2] In the *Vita Hippocratis* attributed to Soranus there is no mention of a Praxithea, and Hippocrates' mother is said to be Phainarete.

ἐνθείᾳ φύσει κεχρημένος καὶ τοσοῦτον ὑπερβεβηκὼς τῇ τῆς ψυχῆς εὐφυΐᾳ τοὺς προγόνους, ὅσον διενήνοχεν αὐτῶν καὶ τῇ τῆς τέχνης ἀρετῇ. καθαίρει δὲ οὐ θηρίων μὲν γένος, θηριωδῶν δὲ νοσημάτων καὶ ἀγρίων πολλὴν γῆν καὶ θάλατταν διασπείρων πανταχοῦ ὥσπερ ὁ Τριπτόλεμος τὰ τῆς Δήμητρος σπέρματα τὰ τοῦ Ἀσκληπιοῦ βοηθήματα.

τοιγαροῦν ἐνδικώτατα καὶ αὐτὸς ἀνιέρευται πολλαχοῦ τῆς γῆς ἠξίωταί τε τῶν αὐτῶν Ἡρακλεῖ τε καὶ Ἀσκληπιῷ ὑπὸ Ἀθηναίων δωρεῶν. αὐτὸν μετάπεμψαι κελεύων ἀργύριον καὶ χρυσίον, ὅσον ἂν βούληται, δώσειν αὐτῷ. οὗτος γὰρ ἐπίσταται οὐχ ἕνα τρόπον τῆς ἰήσιος τοῦ πάθους, οὗτος πατὴρ ὑγείας, οὗτος σωτήρ, οὗτος ἀκεσώδυνος, οὗτος ἁπλῶς ἡγεμὼν τῆς θεοπρεποῦς ἐπιστήμης. ἔρρωσο.

316 3. Βασιλεὺς βασιλέων μέγας Ἀρταξέρξης Ὑστάνῃ Ἑλλησπόντου ὑπάρχῳ χαίρειν·

Ἱπποκράτους ἰητροῦ Κῴου ἀπὸ Ἀσκληπιοῦ γεγονότος καὶ ἐς ἐμὲ κλέος ἀφῖκται τέχνης. δὸς οὖν αὐτῷ χρυσὸν ὁπόσον ἂν βούληται, καὶ τὰ ἄλλα χύδην ὧν σπανίζει, καὶ πέμπε πρὸς ἡμέας. ἔσται γὰρ Περσέων ἰσότιμος τοῖς ἀρίστοις. καὶ εἴ τις ἐστὶν ἄλλος ἀνὴρ κατ' Εὐρώπην ἀγαθός, φίλον οἴκῳ βασιλέως τίθεσο μὴ φειδόμενος ὄλβου. ἄνδρας γὰρ εὑρεῖν δυναμένους τι κατὰ συμβουλὴν οὐ ῥηΐδιον. ἔρρωσο.

4. Ὑστάνης Ἱπποκράτει ἰητρῷ ἀπὸ Ἀσκληπιοῦ γεγονότι χαίρειν·

Βασιλεὺς μέγας Ἀρταξέρξης σου χρῄζων ἔπεμψε πρὸς ἡμέας ὑπάρχους κελεύων σοι ἀργύριον καὶ χρυσὸν καὶ τὰ ἄλλα χύδην, ὧν σπανίζεις καὶ ὅσα βούλει, διδόναι καὶ πέμπειν πρὸς ἑωυτὸν ἐν τάχει. ἔσεσθαι γὰρ Περσέων τοῖς ἀρίστοις ἰσότιμον. σὺ οὖν παραγίνου ξυντόμως. ἔρρωσο.

---

1 ἐνθείᾳ: θείᾳ bO ἐνθέῳ U ὑπερβέβηκεν b (corr. b^2) εὐγενείᾳ O ‖ 3 νοσημάτων: σωμάτων O ‖ 4 θάλασσαν O τὰ: τὰ μετὰ V μετὰ correctum in τὰ M ‖ 5 τὰ om. V ‖ 6 οὗτος bO ἀνιέρευται: ba νϊέρευται V ἀνιέρωται Ud ἀνιερ ~ται M (dixerat ἀνιερεῦται) ἀνηγόρευται c ‖ 7 $τε^I$: δὲ O $τε^{II}$ om. O ‖ 9 οὕτω M γὰρ om. O ‖ 11 ἔρρωσο om. O

3. Mss. p^1p^2MUVbOφ 12 ἐπάρχῳ p^1 ‖ 14-15 κλέος τέχνης ἀφῖκ. φ ‖ 15 τέχνης om., add. superscr., p^1 διδοὺς φ χρυσὸν: O χρυσίον MUVb χρυσὸν καὶ ἄργυρον p^1 ὅσον O ‖ 16 ὧν ἂν (ἐὰν p^1) σπανίζῃ p^1φ καὶ om. φ πρὸς: εἰς MU ὁμότιμος φ ἰσότιμος περσῶν O ‖ 17 τοῖς: τοῖ M ante καὶ add. ἀλλὰ φ ἐστὶν om. Oφ ἄλλος ἐστὶν U ἀνὴρ om. V post ἀγαθὸς add. φάνοιτο φ ‖ 17-18 καὶ...τίθεσο om., add. supersc., p^1 ‖ 18 τίθεσο: δίδου οὖν p^1 ποιοῦ O ‖ 18-19 ἄνδρας...ῥηΐδιον om. p^1p^2 ‖ 19 συμβουλίην MUb ἔρρωσο om. p^1Oφ

4. Mss. p^1MUVb 20 Ἱπποκράτους ἰητρῷ...γεγονότος U χαιριν και υγιαινιν p^1 ‖ 21 μέγ. Ἀρτ. om. p^1 ‖ 21-2 ὑπάρχους κελεύων σοι: διδοὺς p^1 ‖ 22 ἀργύριον καὶ χρυσὸν: χρυσὸν καὶ ἄργυρον ὅποσον ἐὰν βούλει p^1 καὶ χρυσὸν: τε καὶ χρυσίον b ὧν σπανίζεις: ὧν ἐὰν σπανίζῃς p^1 ‖ 3-5 καὶ ὅσα...ἰσότιμον om. p^1

employing his divine nature, and surpassing his forebears in the natural quality of his soul by as much as he has surpassed them in scientific excellence. He cleanses the earth and sea over wide areas, not of wild beasts but of beastly wild diseases, and as Triptolemus sowed everywhere the seeds of Demeter, he sows the cures of Asclepius.

Whence justly he has been given divine honors widely on earth and is accorded the same gifts as are Heracles and Asclepius by the Athenians.[1] Do send for him; and direct that he be given all the gold and silver that he wants. For he knows not just a single manner of healing the affection, he is the father of health, savior, soother of pain. In short he is leader in the divine science. Be well!

3. King of Kings, great Artaxerxes to Hystanes, governor of the Hellespont. Greetings.

The fame of the science of the physician, Hippocrates of Cos, descendant of Asclepius, has reached even to me. Give him all the gold he wants, and in abundance all else that he lacks, and send him to me. He will have honor comparable with Persian nobles. And if there is any other good man in Europe, make him a friend to the King's house, sparing no expense. Finding men who have any capacity for advising is not easy. Be well!

4. Hystanes to the physician Hippocrates, descended from Asclepius. Greetings.

The Great King Artaxerxes, desiring you, sent subordinates to me and bade me give you silver and gold and abundantly all else you want and need and bade me send you to him quickly. You will be honored equally with the foremost of Persians. Please come immediately. Be well!

---

[1] The writer asserts that the Athenians accorded Hippocrates the worship appropriate to a hero. He appears to exaggerate the statements in the *Presbeutikos*,*Epibomios*, and *Decree*, where it is said that Hippocrates was initiated into the mysteries at public expense. We do recall, however, that in the *Presbeutikos* Hippocrates' ancestor Fawn is said to have been the recipient of public sacrifice after his death (below, p. 115). Heroization and worship of Hippocrates is not elsewhere part of the tradition, the nearest thing to it being the statement in the Pseudo-Soranus *Vita Hippocratis* that Hippocrates' birthday was celebrated on Cos. The peculiar exaggerations of this letter support the inference that letters 1 and 2 were later additions to the letter group. The terminology at the end of the letter, "savior", etc., is like that used in addresses to Asclepius generally.

5. Ἱπποκράτης ἰητρὸς Ὑστάνῃ Ἑλλησπόντου ὑπάρχῳ χαίρειν.

Πέμπε ἐς βασιλέα ὡς τάχος ὅτι καὶ προσφορῇ καὶ ἐσθῆτι καὶ οἰκήσει καὶ πάσῃ τῇ ἐς βίον ἀρκεούσῃ οὐσίῃ χρέομαι καὶ Περσέων ὄλβῳ οὐ θέλῳ ἐπαύρασθαι οὐδὲ παύειν βαρβάρους ἀνθρώπους νούσων, ἐχθροὺς ἐόντας Ἑλλήνων.

4α. Ὑστάνης Ἱπποκράτει ἰητρῷ Ἀσκληπιαδῶν ὄντι ἀπογόνῳ χαίρειν.

Ἣν ἔπεμψε βασιλεὺς ἐπιστολὴν σέο χρῄζων ἔπεμψά σοι. γράψον οὖν πρὸς ταῦτα ἵνα κατὰ τάχος πρὸς βασιλέα πέμψω. ἔρρωσο.

5α. Ἱπποκράτης ἰητρὸς Ὑστάνῃ Ἑλλησπόντου ὑπάρχῳ χαίρειν.

Πρὸς τὴν ἐπιστολὴν ἣν ἔπεμψας φάμενος παρὰ βασιλέως ἀφῖχθαι, πέμπε
318 βασιλεῖ, ἃ λέγω, γράφων ὅτι τάχος, διότι καὶ προσφορῇ | καὶ ἐσθῆτι καὶ
οἰκήσει καὶ πάσῃ τῇ ἐς βίον ἀρκεούσῃ οὐσίῃ χρεόμεθα. Περσέων δὲ ὄλβου οὔ
μοι θέμις ἐπαύρασθαι οὐδὲ βαρβάρους ἄνδρας νούσων παύειν ἐχθροὺς
ὑπάρχοντας Ἑλλήνων. ἔρρωσο.

6. Ἱπποκράτης Δημητρίῳ ὑγιαίνειν·

Βασιλεὺς Περσέων ἡμέας μεταπέμπεται οὐκ εἰδὼς ὅτι λόγος ἐμοὶ σοφίης χρυσοῦ πλέον δύναται. ἔρρωσο.

6α. Ἱπποκράτης Γοργίᾳ τῷ φιλτάτῳ πλεῖστα χαίρειν καὶ ὑγιαίνειν·

Βασιλεὺς ὁ Περσέων μεταπέμψασθαι ἡμέας ἐβουλήθη ἐπὶ χρυσῷ τε καὶ ἀργυρῷ πανπλήθει ἀγνόων ὅτι λόγος ἐμὸς σοφίῃ κεχρημένος χρυσοῦ μέζονα δύναμιν ἔχει.

---

ante quintam epistulam ὁ δὲ γενναῖος τηρήσας τὸ τῆς τέχνης ἀξίωμα καὶ τὸ πρὸς τοὺς Ἕλληνας φιλόστοργον ἀντεφώνησεν γράψας τὸν τρόπον τοῦτον· addidit p^1 ante quintam epistulam ἀντίγραφος Ἱπποκράτους πρὸς Ὑστάνην add. φ

5. Mss. p^1p^2(apparet post 5a)O(=acd)φ 1 ἰητρὸς om. p^2 post ἰητρὸς add. ὑπὸ γένους Ἀσκληπιαδέων p^1 ἐπάρχῳ p^1 ἱππάρχῳ c Ἑλλησπ. om p^1 Ἑλλησπ. post ὑπάρχῳ O ‖ 2 ἐς βασιλέα:]σιλέως p^2 ‖ 3 ἀρκεύσῃ p^1 συνουσίῃ p^2 περιουσίῃ φ οὐσίῃ ante ἀρκεούσῃ O]εσθαι (fort. χρέεσθαι) p^2 καὶ Περσέων ὄλβῳ: ὄλβου δὲ Περσῶν φ οὐ θέλῳ: [μοι θέ]μις p^2 ἐπάρασθαι φ ‖ 4 παῦσαι φ ἀνθρώπους: ἄνδρας p^2 ἐόντας: ὑπάρχοντας p^2

4a. Mss. p^1(marg.)p^2p^3Oφ 6 Ὑστ. Ἑλλησπόντου ὑπάρχος p^3 ἰητρῷ om. O post ἰητρῷ add. κῴῳ p^1φ ‖ 7 ὁ βασ. O post βασ. add. μέγας p^3 πέπομφά p^1φ ‖ 7-8 γράψον...ταῦτα om. p^1p^3 ‖ 8 ταύτην O ἵνα [τὴν σὴν] ἀπόφ[ασ]ιν κατὰ p^3 κατὰ τάχος ἵνα O πρὸς βασιλέα om. p^2φ πρὸς: ἐς p^1

5a. Mss. p^2p^3MUVb (p^3 is too tattered in this letter to give secure information) 9 ἰητρὸς om. p^2V ‖ 10 τὴν ἣν ἔπεμψας ἐπιστ. V ‖ 11 ἃ λέγω γράφων: λέγων γράφω p^2 ἃ ἐγὼ γράφω b ὅτι τάχος om. p^2 διότι: ὅτι p^2 ‖ 12 ante βίον add. τὸν b συνουσίῃ p^2 χρεώμεθα MU χρέομαι p^2 Περσέων δὲ ὄλβου: καὶ ὄλβου Περσέων p^2

6. Mss. MUVbφcd 15 post Δημ. add. βασιλεῖ b χαίρειν c ‖ 16 ἐμῆς σοφίης c

6a. Apparet unice in p^1 20 λογσο p^1

5. Hippocrates the physician to Hystanes, governor of the Hellespont. Greetings.

Send back to the King as quickly as possible that I have enough food, clothing, shelter and all substance sufficient for life, and I am unwilling to enjoy Persian opulence or to save Persians from disease, since they are enemies of the Greeks. Be well!

4a.[1] Hystanes to the physician Hippocrates, who is descended from the Asclepiads. Greetings.

I have sent to you the letter which the king sent in his desire for you. Write a response to it please, so that I can send it to the king quickly. Be well!

5a.[2] Hippocrates the physician to Hystanes, governor of the Hellespont. Greetings.

In response to the letter you sent which you said came from the King, write to the King and send him as quickly as possible what I say: I have enough food, clothing, shelter and all substance sufficient for life. It is not proper that I should enjoy Persian opulence or save Persians from disease, since they are enemies of the Greeks. Be well!

6. Hippocrates to Demetrius. Health.

The King of the Persians has summoned me, in ignorance that for me wisdom's message is more powerful than gold. Be well!

6a.[3] Hippocrates to his dearest Gorgias. Best of greetings and health.

The King of the Persians wanted to summon me on condition of abundant gold and silver, in his ignorance that my reasoning which deals in wisdom has more power than gold.

---

[1] This form of letter 4 appears in one Renaissance manuscript and in the ancient papyrus manuscripts from Egypt, showing that there were distinct versions as early as the first century A. D. 4 and 4a both appear in our earliest papyrus (P. Oxy. 1184). 4a seems to be the version most properly answered by letter 5, and referred to by letter 7.

[2] In P. Oxy. 1184 letter 5 is introduced by the following: "But the excellent man, vigilant for the reputation of his science and for his love of the Greeks wrote in reply in the following manner:" The form implies an early presentation of these brief letters which offered introductory descriptions of them.

[3] This version of letter 6 appears only in P. Oxy. 1184. The addressee is presumably the sophist Gorgias whom the Life of Hippocrates by "Soranus" describes as Hippocrates' teacher.

7. βασιλεῖ βασιλέων τῷ ἐμῷ μεγάλῳ δεσπότῃ Ἀρταξέρξῃ Ὑστάνης Ἑλλησπόντου ὕπαρχος χαίρειν·

Ἣν ἔπεμψας ἐπιστολὴν λέγων πέμψαι Ἱπποκράτει, ἰητρῷ Κῴῳ ἀπὸ Ἀσκληπιαδῶν γεγονότι, ἔπεμψα, καὶ παρ' αὐτοῦ δὲ ἐκομισάμην ἀπόκρισιν ἣν γράψας ἔδωκε καὶ ἐκέλευσεν εἰς σὸν οἶκον πέμπειν. φέροντα οὖν ἀπέστειλά σοι Φενακάσβην. διευτύχει. ἔρρωσο.

8. Βασιλεὺς βασιλέων μέγας Ἀρταξέρξης Κῴοις τάδε λέγει·

Δότε ἐμοῖς ἀγγέλοις Ἱπποκράτην ἰητρὸν κακοὺς τρόπους ἔχοντα καὶ εἰς ἐμὲ καὶ εἰς Πέρσας ἀσελγαίνοντα. εἰ δὲ μή, γνώσεσθε καὶ τῆς πρώτης ἁμαρτίας τιμωρίαν τίσοντες. δηϊώσας γὰρ τὴν ὑμετέραν πόλιν καὶ νῆσον κατασπάσας εἰς πέλαγος ποιήσω μηδὲ εἰς τὸν ἐπίλοιπον χρόνον γνῶναι, εἰ ἦν ἐπὶ τούτῳ τῷ τόπῳ νῆσος ἢ πόλις Κῶ.

9. Ἀπόκρισις Κῴων.

320 Ἔδοξε τῷ δάμῳ ἀποκρίνασθαι τοῖς παρὰ Ἀρταξέρξου ἀγγέλοις, | ὅτι Κῷοι οὐδὲν ἀνάξιον πράξουσιν οὔτε Μέροπος οὔτε Ἡρακλέους οὔτε Ἀσκληπιοῦ, ὧν ἕνεκε πάντες οἱ πολῖται οὐ δώσουσιν Ἱπποκράτεα, οὐδὲ εἰ μέλλοιεν ὀλέθρῳ τῷ κακίστῳ ἀπολεῖσθαι. καὶ γὰρ Δαρείου καὶ Ξέρξου ἀπὸ πατέρων ἐπιστολὰς γραψάντων γαῖαν καὶ ὕδωρ αἰτεόντων οὐκ ἔδωκεν ὁ δᾶμος ὁρέων αὐτοὺς ὁμοίως τοῖς ἄλλοις ἀνθρώπους θνατοὺς ἐόντας ἐπ' αὐτοὺς ἰόντας. καὶ νῦν τὰν αὐτὰν ἀπόκρισιν διδοῖ· ἀπὸ Κῴων ἀναχωρεῖτε, ὅτι Ἱπποκράτην οὐ δίδοντι ἔκδοτον. ἀπαγγέλλετε οὖν αὐτῷ οἱ ἄγγελοι, ὅτι οὐδ' οἱ θεοὶ ἀμελήσουσιν ἁμέων.

10. Ἀβδηριτῶν ἡ βουλὴ καὶ ὁ δῆμος Ἱπποκράτει χαίρειν·

Κινδυνεύεται τὰ μέγιστα τῇ πόλει νῦν, Ἱππόκρατες· ἀνὴρ ἡμετέρων, ὃς καὶ τῷ παρόντι χρόνῳ καὶ τῷ μέλλοντι αἰεὶ κλέος ἠλπίζετο τῇ πόλει,

---

7-9. Mss. MUVbφcd 1 ἐμῷ om. V ‖ 1-2 βασιλεῖ...χαίρειν: γράφη Ὑστάνους πρὸς Ἀρταξέρξην φ ‖ 3 Ἣν ἔπεμψας: ἀνέπεμψας U ‖ 4 δὲ om. φ ‖ 5 ἐκέλευεν V ἠξίωσεν φ σὸν: ὃν M ‖ 6 ἀπέσταλκα φ φέροντα... ἔρρωσο om. c Φενακάσβην: scripsi φενακηνάσβην φ φάναι γυμνάσβην UMb γυμνάσβην Vd δι' εὐτύχη φ ἔρρωσο om. b ‖ 8 ante ἐμοῖς add. τοῖς φ post ἔχοντα add. καὶ εἰς ὑμᾶς φ ‖ 9 τῆς πρώτης: πρὸ τῆς φ ‖ 10 τίσαντες φ ὑμῶν τὴν πόλιν καὶ τὴν νῆσον φ ‖ 11 τὸ λοιπὸν χρόνον φ γνωσθῆναι φ γνώσεσθαι M (corr. M^2) ‖ 12 ἐπὶ: ἐν φ ἔτι ἐν MUd κῴῳν φ ‖ 13 Κῴων om. φ ‖ 14 τῷ δάμῳ: τῇ πόλει φ ἀποκρίνεσθαι M^2 περὶ φ ‖ 15 ἀντάξιον VM (corr. M^2) πραξαντες φ Μέροπος: Ἄρεος φ ‖ 16 ὧν...πολῖται: ὠνοντί πάντες οἱ λοιποὶ φ οὐ: οὔτε MUc (corr. in οὐ) d Ἱπποκράτην φb ‖ 17 μέλλει U ante ὀλέθρῳ add ἄρτι. φ τῶν b ἀπολέσθαι V ‖ 18 πάτρων φ ante γαῖαν add καὶ b γαῖαν om. φ ‖ 18-19 οὐκ ἔδωκεν αἰτούντων φ ‖ 19 ἀνθρώποις MUbφc θνητοὺς Ucd θανάτους MVb (marg.) θνάτους M^2 et in marg. γρ. καὶ θνητοὺς ‖ 19-20 θνατ. ἐόντ. om. bφ ‖ 20 ἐπ' αὐτοὺς ἰόντας: om. c ἀπ' αὐτοὺς ὄντας φ τὰν αὐτὰν: τὰν αὖ U τᾶν αὐτᾶν c ἀπόκρισιν διδοῖ om. MUVφcd ‖ 21 ἀποχωρεῖτε Uc ἀποχωρεῖται Md ἀναχωρεῖτε ὅτι om. φ Ἱπποκράτης U δίδονται MUVcd διδόντην φ ‖ 21-2 ἀπαγγελόντων δὲ αὐτῶν οἱ φ ‖ 22 post ἁμέων add. δόντι Ἱπποκράτεα ἁμέων Md δόντων Ἱπποκράτεα U μὴ δόντες Ἱπποκράτεα ὑμῖν c

10. Mss. MUVbcd 24 κινδυνεύει cb (corr. b^2) νυνί U ante ἡμετ. add. τῶν bc ἡμέτερον U ‖ 25 ἠλπίζετο: ἐφάνη c

7. Hystanes, viceroy of the Hellespont to Artaxerxes, King of Kings, my great lord. Greetings.

I forwarded the letter which you sent with orders to send it to Hippocrates, physician of the Coans, born of the Asclepiads, and from him got a response which he wrote, gave to me, and bade me send to your house. I have sent Phenakaspes to bring you the letter. May you have good fortune. Be well![1]

8. King of Kings, great Artaxerxes, says the following to the Coans:

Give to my messengers Hippocrates, a physician of bad character who has been insolent toward me and toward the Persians. If you do not, you will learn that you will pay the penalty for initiating the wrongdoing. I will destroy your city, drag the island into the sea, and make it so that it will not even be known in time to come that there was an island or city of Cos in that spot.

9. The Coans' Answer:[2]

It was voted by the people to answer the messengers from Artaxerxes that the Coans will do nothing unworthy of Merops or Heracles or Asclepius, wherefore the citizens all together will not give up Hippocrates, not even if they should be going to die the worst of deaths. Indeed, when Darius and Xerxes wrote letters demanding earth and water from our fathers, the people did not give it, seeing that those who were coming against them were mortal men like everyone else. Now the people give the same answer. Depart from the Coans because they are not going to deliver up Hippocrates. Inform him, messengers, that neither will the gods be unconcerned with us.[3]

10. The Council and the people of Abdera to Hippocrates. Greetings.

Our city is now in great peril, Hippocrates. That man of all our citizens who we always expected would be the fame of our city/in the present and future

---

[1] Phenakaspes is perhaps a mock Persian name on the model of such names as Hystaspes (Hdt.1.183.3, etc.). Phenakizo means "cheat" in Greek; phenake is false hair.

[2] The Coans' Decree is in a literary Doric which in large part corresponds with the dialect used by formal Coan decrees, that is to say, the "Doric koine" used in the Doric communities of the Aegean region after the fifth century B.C. See Carl D. Buck's description, *The Greek Dialects* (Chicago: 1955) 173-80, and the Coan Decree on procedures of sacrifice which he gives as an example, pp. 302-4 (The same decree appears as P-H 37, and number 43 of Felix Solmsen, *Inscriptiones Graecae ad Inlustrandas Dialectos Selectae*, 2nd edition by Ernest Fraenkel (Leipzig: 1930).

[3] The readings of Mss. MUd suggest that one version of the letter ended "Neither will the gods be unmindful of us if we give him up."

μηδὲν νῦν ὧδε, πάντες θεοί, φθονηθείη, οὗτος, ὑπὸ πολλῆς τῆς κατεχούσης αὐτὸν σοφίης νενόσηκεν, ὥστε φόβος οὐχ ὁ τυχών, ἂν φθαρῇ Δημόκριτος τὸν λογισμόν, ἐόντως δὴ τὴν πόλιν ἡμέων Ἀβδηριτῶν καταλειφθήσεσθαι. ἐκλαθόμενος γὰρ ἁπάντων καὶ ἑωυτοῦ καὶ πρότερον, ἐγρηγορὼς καὶ ἡμέρην καὶ νύκτα, γελῶν ἕκαστα σμικρὰ καὶ μεγάλα, καὶ μηδὲν οἰόμενος εἶναι τὸν βίον ὅλον διατελεῖ. γαμεῖ τις, ὁ δὲ ἐμπορεύεται, ὁ δὲ δημηγορεῖ, ἄλλος ἄρχει, πρεσβεύει, χειροτονεῖται, νοσεῖ, τέτρωται, |
322 τέθνηκεν· ὁ δὲ πάντα γελᾷ, τοὺς μὲν κατηφεῖς τε καὶ σκυθρωπούς, τοὺς δὲ χαίροντας ὁρῶν. ζητεῖ δὲ ὁ ἀνὴρ καὶ περὶ τῶν ἐν Ἅιδου καὶ γράφει ταῦτα καὶ εἰδώλων φησὶ πλήρη τὸν ἠέρα εἶναι καὶ ὀρνέων φωνὰς ὠτακουστεῖ· καὶ πολλάκις νύκτωρ ἐξαναστὰς μόνος ἡσυχῇ ᾠδὰς ᾄδοντι ἔοικεν· καὶ ἀποδημεῖν ἐνίοτε λέγει ἐς τὴν ἀπειρίην καὶ Δημοκρίτους εἶναι ὁμοίους ἑωυτῷ ἀναριθμήτους· καὶ συνδιεφθορὼς τῇ γνώμῃ τὸ χρῶμα ζῇ.

2. ταῦτα φοβούμεθα, Ἱππόκρατες, ταῦτα ταραττόμεθα. ἀλλὰ σῷζε καὶ ταχὺς ἐλθὼν νουθέτησον ἡμέων τὴν πατρίδα. οὐκ ἂν ἁμάρτοις οὔτε δόξης τῆς ἐπ' αὐτῷ περισωθέντι οὔτε χρημάτων οὔτε παιδείης. καίτοι τὰ παιδείης πολλῷ σοι βελτίω τῶν τῆς τύχης. ἀλλ' οὖν καὶ ταῦτα συχνὰ παρ' ἡμέων καὶ ἄφθονα γενήσεται, τῆς γὰρ Δημοκρίτεω ψυχῆς. ἀλλ' οὐδ' εἰ χρυσὸς ἂν ἔῃ, ἡ πόλις ἀντάξια βουλήσιος οὐδ' ὁτιοῦν ἀφυστερήσεται. τοὺς νόμους ἡμέων δοκοῦμεν νοσεῖν, Ἱππόκρατες, τοὺς νόμους παρακόπτειν. ἴθι θεραπεύσων, ἀνδρῶν φέριστε, ἄνδρα ἀρίδηλον, οὐκ ἰητρός, ἀλλὰ κτίστης ἐὼν ὅλης τῆς Ἰωνίης, περιβάλλων ἡμῖν ἱερώτερον τεῖχος. πόλιν, οὐκ ἄνδρα θεραπεύσεις, βουλὴν δὲ νοσοῦσαν καὶ κινδυνεύουσαν ἀποκλεισθῆναι μέλλεις ἀνοιγνύναι. αὐτὸς νομοθέτης, αὐτὸς δικαστής, αὐτὸς ἄρχων, αὐτὸς σωτὴρ καὶ τούτων τεχνίτης ἀφίξει. ταῦτά σε προσδοκῶμεν, Ἱππόκρατες, ταῦτα καὶ γένοιο ἐλθών. μία πόλεων οὐκ
324 ἄσημος, μᾶλλον δὲ | ἡ Ἑλλὰς ὅλη δεῖταί σου φυλάξαι σῶμα σοφίης. αὐτὴν δὲ δόκει παιδείαν πρεσβεύειν πρὸς σὲ τῆς παρακοπῆς ταύτης ἀπαλλαγῆναι δεομένην. ξυγγενὲς μὲν οὖν, ὡς ἔοικε, πᾶσι σοφία, τοῖσι δ' ἐγγυτέρω κεχωρηκόσιν αὐτῆς ὥσπερ ὑμῖν καὶ μάλα πλέον. εὖ ἴσθι, χαριεῖ καὶ τῷ μέλλοντι αἰῶνι μὴ προεκλιπεῖν Δημόκριτον ἧς ἐλπίζει προτέρησιν ἀληθείης. σὺ γὰρ Ἀσκληπιῷ προσπέπλεξαι γένος καὶ τέχνην,

---

1 μὴ δὲ Vbc ὧδε: ὅδε U δὲ bc ante πάντες add. ὦ Ubc ‖ 2 ante Δημ. add. ὁ d ‖ 2-3 τὸν λογισμὸν Δημόκριτος MUbcd ‖ 3 ἐόντως δὴ: οὕτως νῦν d ‖ 4 καὶ ante πρότερον om. Vbc ‖ 5 νύκτα καὶ ἥμ. MUd γελῶν: λέγων M ‖ 7 ἄλλος...πρεσβεύει om. c post χειροτονεῖται add. ἀποχειροτονεῖται b post τέτρωται add. τὸ πᾶν bc ‖ 8 γελᾷ πάντα MUd τε om. Vbc ‖ 11 ὠτακουστεῖν MUd ‖ 12 καὶ ante Δημ. bis V post Δημ. add. πολλοὺς bc ‖ 13 σὺν διεφθορὰς U in marg. γρ. συνδιεφθορὼς τὸ σῶμα τῇ ψυχῇ ζῇ M ‖ 14 post ταῦτα add. δὴ bc γὰρ ἀττώμεθα V ‖ 15 νουθετήσων MUd post πατρίδα add. μὴ δὴ ἡμᾶς ἀποβαλῇς καὶ γὰρ οὐδὲ ἀποβλητοί ἐσμεν. ἡ (καὶ H) ἐν ὑμῖν μαρτυρία κεῖται cH(marg.) ‖ 16 τῆς om. b ‖ 19 ἂν ἔῃ: scripsi ἦν mss. ἀφυστερήσεται: scripsi ἀφυστερήσαντα MVbc -αντος U -αντι d in marg. γρ. τὸ δοῦλον ουδ' ἀφυστερήσαντας b ‖ 21 θεράπευσον U ἄνδρα ἀρίδηλον om. Vbc ‖ 22 περιβαλὼν Vbc ἱερωτέρως U ‖ 23 θεραπεύεις UV δὲ νοσοῦσαν καὶ: διὰ νόσον Vbc ‖ 24 μέλλοις MUV ἀνυγνῦναι U αὐτὸς[II] om. bc ‖ 25 τούτου c ἀφίξῃ UVbc ‖ 26 post ἐλθὼν add ἅμα, et superscr. add. b πόλεως U ‖ 27 δὲ om. Vbc ‖ 29 πάσῃ U ‖ 30 ἐγγυτέρῳ Mb ἐγγυτέροις U ἡμῖν MUV ‖ 31 χαίρει MU προλιπεῖν V ‖ 32 προτερήσειν bc γένει καὶ τέχνῃ V

(All gods! May it not be begrudged in this way now!), that man has been made ill by the great learning that weighs him down. As a result there is no small fear that if Democritus has lost his reason, the city of us Abderites will be, in truth, left empty. For, previously inattentive to everything, including himself, he is now constantly wakeful night and day, laughs at everything large and small, and thinks life in general is worth nothing. Someone marries, a man engages in trade, a man goes into politics, another takes an office, goes on an embassy, votes, falls ill, is wounded, dies. He laughs at every one of them, whether he sees them downcast and ill-tempered, or happy. The man is investigating things in Hades, and he writes about them, and he says that the air is full of images. He listens to birds' voices. Arising often alone at night he seems to be singing softly. He claims that he goes off sometimes into the boundless and that there are numberless Democrituses like himself. He lives with a complexion as ruined as his reason.

2. These are our fears Hippocrates, this is our perturbation.[1] Save us, come swiftly and bring reason to our land. You would not fail of fame for saving him, nor money, nor learning. And for you, the fruits of learning are far better than what luck brings. But that, too, will come abundantly and ungrudgingly from us. Because it is for the life of Democritus. Not even if it be gold will the city fall the least bit short of the full amount you desire. We seem to have fallen ill in our ways, Hippocrates, have gone insane in our laws. Come, best of men, to heal a man most prominent. Come not as a doctor, but as a founder of all Ionia, casting about us a holy bulwark. You will heal a city, not just a man, and you will open a senate that is sick and in danger of being closed up. You yourself will come as lawgiver, yourself as judge, yourself as ruler, yourself as savior and craftsman of these things. These things we expect of you, Hippocrates. May you come and be these things. Not just a single city, obscure among cities, but rather all Hellas begs you to protect the very person of wisdom. It seems as though learning herself is ambassador to you, begging to be relieved of this madness. Wisdom is a thing akin to everyone but even more to those who have come nearest her, like you. Be certain that it will be a joy to posterity also if Democritus does not leave off before that truth in which he hopes for excellence. You have been bound to Asclepius in family and in science.

[1] ταραττόμεθα: The Abderites use terminology which indicates that they need the *ataraxia* which Epicurean philosophy brings. The early Cynics used ἀπάθεια along with αὐτάρκεια το describe their detachment from mundane concerns.

ὁ δὲ Ἡρακλέους ἐστὶν ἀδελφιδοῦς, ἀφ' οὗ Ἄβδηρος, ὥς που πυνθάνῃ πάντως, ᾧ ἐπώνυμος ἡ πόλις. ὥστε κἀκείνῳ χάρις ἡ Δημοκρίτου γένοιτ' ἂν ἴησις. ὁρῶν οὖν, ὦ Ἱππόκρατες, ἐς ἀναισθησίαν ἀπορρέοντα καὶ δῆμον καὶ ἄνδρα ἀρίσημον, σπεῦδε πρὸς ἡμέας, δεόμεθα. φεῦ, ὡς καὶ τὰ ἀγαθὰ περισσεύσαντα νοῦσοι τυγχάνουσιν. ὁ Δημόκριτος γὰρ ὅσον ἐρρώσθη πρὸς ἄκρα σοφίης, ἴσα κινδυνεύει νῦν ἀποπληξίᾳ διανοίας καὶ ἠλιθιότητι κεκακῶσθαι. οἱ δ' ἄλλοι ὅσοι πολλοὶ Ἀβδηριτῶν μείναντες ἐν ἀπαιδευσίῃ τόν γε κοινὸν κατέχουσι νοῦν, ἀλλὰ νῦν γε φρονιμώτεροι νόσον σοφοῦ κρίνειν οἱ πρὶν ἄφρονες. ἴθι οὖν μετὰ Ἀσκληπιοῦ πατρός, ἴθι μετὰ Ἡρακλέους θυγατρὸς Ἠπιόνης, ἴθι μετὰ παίδων τῶν ἐπὶ Ἴλιον στρατευσαμένων, ἴθι νῦν παιώνια νούσου φέρων ἄκη. εὐκαρπήσαι δὲ γῆ ῥίζας καὶ βοτάνας, ἀλεξιφάρμακα μανίης ἄνθη. σχεδὸν οὐδέποτε γονιμώτερον εὐφορήσουσιν οὔτε γῆ οὔτε ὀρῶν ἀκρώρειαι ἢ νῦν Δημοκρίτῳ τὰ πρὸς τὴν ὑγείην. ἔρρωσο.

11. Ἱπποκράτης Ἀβδηριτῶν βουλῇ καὶ δήμῳ χαίρειν·

326 Ὁ πολίτης ὑμέων Ἀμελησαγόρης ἦλθεν ἐς Κῶ, καὶ ἔτυχε τότ' | ἐοῦσα τῆς ῥάβδου ἡ ἀνάληψις ἐν ἐκείνῃ τῇ ἡμέρῃ καὶ ἐτήσιος ἑορτή, ὡς ἴστε, πανήγυρις ἡμῖν, καὶ πομπὴ πολυτελὴς ἐς κυπάρισσον, ἣν ἔθος ἀνάγειν τοῖσι τῷ θεῷ προσήκουσι. ἐπεὶ δὲ σπουδάζειν ἐῴκει καὶ ἐκ τῶν λόγων καὶ ἐκ τῆς ὄψιος ὁ Ἀμελησαγόρης, πεισθείς, ὅπερ ἦν, ἐπείγειν τὸ πρῆγμα, ἀνέγνων τε ὑμέων τὴν ἐπιστολὴν καὶ ἐθαύμασα ὅτι περὶ ἑνὸς ἀνθρώπου ὡς εἷς ἄνθρωπος ἡ πόλις θορυβεῖσθε. μακάριοί γε δῆμοι καὶ ὁκόσοι ἴσασι τοὺς ἀγαθοὺς ἄνδρας ἐρύματα ἑωυτῶν καὶ οὐ τοὺς πύργους οὐδὲ τὰ τείχεα, ἀλλὰ σοφῶν ἀνδρῶν σοφὰς γνώμας. ἐγὼ δὲ πειθόμενος τέχνας μὲν εἶναι θεῶν χάριτας, ἀνθρώπους δὲ ἔργα φύσιος, καὶ μὴ νεμεσήσητε, ἄνδρες Ἀβδηρῖται, οὐχ ὑμᾶς δοκέω, ἀλλὰ φύσιν αὐτὴν καλεῖν με ἀνασώσασθαι ποίημα ἑωυτῆς κινδυνεῦον ὑπὸ νούσου διαπεσεῖν. ὥστε πρὸ ὑμέων ἐγὼ νῦν φύσει καὶ θεοῖσιν ὑπακούω νοσέοντα Δημόκριτον ἰήσασθαι, εἰ δὴ καὶ νοῦσός ἐστιν, ἀλλὰ μὴ ἀπάτη συσκιάζεσθε, ὅπερ εὔχομαι. καὶ γένοιτο καὶ πλέον τῆς ἐν ὑμῖν εὐνοίας τε κμήριον καὶ πρὸς ὑπόνοιαν

---

2 ᾧ om. bc Δημοκρίτω U || 3 ὦ om. Vb || 6 ἄκρα corr. in ἄκραν b || 7 ante Ἀβδηριτῶν add. δ' εἰσὶν MVb || 8 γε: τε MUd νῦν γε: μὴν καὶ MU || 9 post πατρὸς add. καὶ πάτρωος (πατραος b) Ἀπόλλωνος bc || 10 Ἡρακλέως U || 11 νῦν om. Vbc παιόνια MVb γρ. καὶ παιῶνις in marg. M εὐκαρπήσαι: scripsi εὐκαρπῆσαι MUVbc εὐκαρπήσει b[2]d || 12 ῥίζαις καὶ βοτάναις Md ῥίζες καὶ βοτάνες U σχεδρὸ U post σχεδὸν add. οὖν bc || 13 ἀκρωτήρια b[2]

11. Mss. p[3](p[2] vix legibilis)MUVbO(=acd) 15 Ἱπποκράτης om. ad Ἱπποκράτους U ante βουλῇ add. τῇ MUbO καὶ om. V ante δήμῳ add τῷ. MUb καὶ δήμῳ χαίρειν om. O || 16 μελισαγόρας O ἧκεν p[3]O ἧς Κῶ U || 17 ἡ ἀνάληψις (ἄναψις a) τῆς ῥάβδου O ἑορτή: ὥρη b om. p[3]O || 18 ἡμῖν om. O πομπη ην[ ]τελεα p[3] πόμπην πολυτελέα b ἣν b ην p[3] ἄγειν O || 19 ἐδώκει U deficit hic p[3] || 20 προσόψιος (-εως c) UMO ἦν: ἐπῆν V || 22 θορυβεῖσθαι MU καὶ om. bO ἴσασι: ἴασις U || 23 ἐρύματα: ἕρματα O ante ἐρύμ. add. καὶ b deficit hic p[2] οὐ τοὺς: αὐτοὺς a || 24 σοφὰς om. sed add. in marg. M γνώμας σοφάς U πείθομαι O || 25 νεμήσητε corr. in νεμήσηται U νῦνεμεσησητε (om. μὴ) V || 26-27 ἐμὲ ἀνασῶσαι O || 27 διαπεσεῖν: διαφθαρῆναι V || 28 νῦν om. O ὑπακούων σπεύδω U || 29 εἴγε δὴ O εἴπερ δὴ MU ante νοῦσος add. τοῦτο MUb συσκιάζεσθαι MUbd || 30 καὶ ante πλέον om. UOM[2] ἡμῖν U

And Asclepius was the nephew of Heracles. From Heracles, as you are perhaps perfectly aware, came Abderos for whom our city is named. So the cure of Democritus would be a kindness to him as well. Seeing our people and a famous man dribbling away to insensibility, hurry to us, we beg. Oh, how even excessive good becomes disease! Democritus, as he had strength for the heights of wisdom, is equally in danger of ruination by a stroke to his mind and by silliness. The other Abderites, many as they are, who remained unlearned, keep the common mind, but, witless before, they now have more wit for judging the disease of a wise man. Come with father Asclepius. Come with Epione, Heracles' daughter. Come with her sons who fought against Troy.[1] Come with Apollo's cures for disease./May the land be fruitful with roots and plants, the flowers that cure madness. Maybe the land and mountaintops will never have borne more productively than now, for Democritus, the plants that heal. Be well!

11. Hippocrates to the Senate and People of Abdera. Greetings.

Your fellow citizen Amelesagoras came to Cos. It chanced to be the day of the Assumption of the Staff, which you know is an annual festival and elaborate procession to the cypress grove customarily led by people related to the god. Because Amelesagoras gave the impression of urgency by his speech and expression, I was convinced (as was the case) that the matter was pressing. I read your letter and found it amazing that you, the whole city, like a single man, were in an uproar about a single man. Blessed are peoples who know that their good men are their defense, not towers and bulwarks, but rather the wise minds of wise men. I, convinced that science is the gift of the gods, and that men are the works of Nature (take no offense, Abderites), believe that not you, but Nature herself is calling me to save her creation which is in danger of crumbling through disease. Hence instead of you I now obey Nature and the gods' command to heal the ailing Democritus, if indeed it is disease and you are not darkly deceived, as I in fact pray. May it be still further testimony of your good will that you were perturbed

---

[1] Epione is wife of Asclepius, mother of Machaon and Podalirius.

ταραχθῆναι. ἀργύριον δέ μοι ἐρχομένῳ οὔτ' ἂν φύσις οὔτ' ἂν θεὸς ὑπόσχοιτο. ὥστε μηδ' ὑμεῖς, ἀνέρες Ἀβδηρῖται, βιάζεσθε, ἀλλ' ἐᾶτε ἐλευθέρης τέχνης ἐλεύθερα καὶ τὰ ἔργα. οἱ δὲ μισθαρνεῦντες δουλεύειν ἀναγκάζουσι τὰς ἐπιστήμας ὥσπερ ἐξανδραποδίζοντες αὐτὰς ἐκ τῆς προτέρης παρρησίης. εἶθ', ὡς εἰκός, καὶ ψεύσαιντο ἂν ὡς περὶ μεγάλης
328 νούσου καὶ ἀρνηθεῖεν ἂν ὡς περὶ | μικρῆς, καὶ οὐκ ἂν ἔλθοιεν ὑποσχόμενοι καὶ πάλιν ἔλθοιεν μὴ κληθέντες. οἰκτρός γε ὁ τῶν ἀνθρώπων βίος, ὅτι δι' ὅλου αὐτοῦ ὡς πνεῦμα χειμέριον ἡ ἀφόρητος φιλαργυρίη διαδέδυκεν, ἐφ' ἣν εἴθε μάλιστα ἅπαντες ἰητροὶ ξυνήεσαν ἀποθεραπεῦσαι χαλεπωτέρην μανίης νοῦσον, ὅτι καὶ μακαρίζεται νοῦσος ἐοῦσα καὶ κακοῦσα. οἶμαι δὲ ἔγωγε καὶ τὰ ψυχῆς νοσήματα πάντα μανίας εἶναι σφοδρὰς ἐμποιούσας δόξας τινὰς καὶ φαντασίας τῷ λογισμῷ, ὧν ὁ δι' ἀρετῆς ὑποκαθαρθεὶς ὑγιάζεται. ἐγὼ δὲ εἰ πλουτεῖν ἐξ ἅπαντος ἐβουλόμην, ὦ ἄνδρες Ἀβδηρῖται, οὐκ ἂν εἵνεκε δέκα ταλάντων διέβαινον πρὸς ὑμέας, ἀλλ' ἐπὶ τὸν μέγαν ἠρχόμην Περσέων βασιλέα, ἔνθα πόλεις ὅλαι προσῆσαν τῆς ἐξ ἀνθρώπων εὐδαιμονίης γεγεμισμέναι. ἰώμην δ' ἂν τὸν ἐκεῖσε λοιμόν, ἀλλ' ἀπηρνησάμην ἐχθρὴν Ἑλλάδι χώρην ἐλευθερῶσαι κακῆς νούσου κἀγὼ τό γε ἐπ' ἐμοὶ καταναυμαχῶν τοὺς βαρβάρους. εἶχον δ' ἂν αἰσχύνην τὸν παρὰ βασιλέως πλοῦτον καὶ πατρίδος ἐχθρὴν περιουσίην, περιεκείμην δ' ἂν αὐτὰ ὡς ἐλέπολις τῆς Ἑλλάδος ὑπάρχων. οὐκ ἔστι πλοῦτος τὸ πανταχόθεν χρηματίζεσθαι. μεγάλα γὰρ ἱερὰ τῆς ἀρετῆς ἐστιν ἐπὶ δικαιοσύνην, οὐκ ὀρυσσόμενα ἀλλ' ἐμφανέα ἐόντα. ἦ οὐκ οἴεσθε ἴσον ἁμάρτημα σῴζειν πολεμίους καὶ φίλους μισθοῦ; ἀλλ' οὐχ ὧδε ἔχει τὰ ἡμέτερα, ὦ δῆμε. οὐ καρποῦμαι δὲ νούσους οὐδὲ δι' εὐχῆς ἤκουσα τὴν Δημοκρίτεω παράκρουσιν, ὅς, εἴτε ὑγιαίνει, φίλος ἔσται, εἴτε νοσεῖ,
330 θεραπευθεὶς πλέον ὑπάρξει. πυν|θάνομαι δὲ αὐτὸν ἐμβριθέα καὶ στερρὸν τὰ ἤθεα καὶ τῆς ὑμετέρης πόλεως ἐόντα κόσμον. ἔρρωσθε.

12. Ἱπποκράτης Φιλοποίμενι χαίρειν·

Οἱ τὴν τῆς πόλιος ἐπιστολὴν ἀποδόντες μοι πρέσβεις καὶ τεὴν ἀπέδοσαν· ἥσθην τε κάρτα καὶ ξεινίην ὑπισχνεομένου σέο καὶ τὴν ἑτέρην

---

1 οὔτε θεὸς O ‖ 2 ἀνέρες: om. bO ante Ἀβδ. add. ὦ b βιάζεσθαι MU ‖ 3 καὶ om. O μισθαργεύοντες VM(corr. M^2) ‖ 6 ἂν om. b ‖ 7 ante γε add. δέ b^2 ‖ 8 ὡς: ὥσπερ b διαδέδοικεν M διαβέβηκεν V ‖ 9 μάλιστα: μᾶλλον bO ξυνήεσαν: ξυνελθόντες MU συνίεσαν d post ξυνήεσαν add. ἐλθόντες Vb (ἠθέλησαν in marg. add. b post ἀποθεραπεῦσαι) ‖ 10 νοῦσος ἐοῦσα: νοσέουσα O κακοῦσα mut. in κακὴ οὖσα b^2 ‖ 11 ante ψυχῆς add. τῆς VO μανίης σφοδρᾶς εἶναι ἐμποιούσης O ‖ 12 τῶν λογισμῶν a ἀποκαθαρθεὶς bad ‖ 14 δώδεκα U ‖ 15 ἐρχόμενος O προσήεσαν M προσίεσαν U παρῆσαν V ‖ 16 εὐδαιμονίης: εὐτυχίης O δ' om. O ἐκεῖ O ἐκεῖσαι U post λοιμόν add. αὐτῶν bdM^2 (in marg.) αὐτὸν U ἀνιῶν ac ‖ 18 γε: μὲν O κατεναυμάχουν UM^2 καταναυμαχῶ O ‖ 13 παρὰ om. O ‖ 20 ἐλεπόλεις M ἔστι: ἔστιν οὖν b ‖ 22 ἐστιν om. O ἐπὶ δικαιοσύνην οὐκ ὀρυσσόμενα: ὑπὸ δικαιοσύνης οὐ κρυπτόμενα MUVb ‖ 23 ante ἴσον add. ὡς b^2 post ἁμάρτημα add. εἶναι MU post φίλους add. ἰᾶσθαι MU post μισθοῦ add. φθείρειν b ὅδε U ‖ 24 ὦ om. ac δῆμαι corr. in δῆμε M δὲ om. sed add. superscr. b ‖ 25 ἔσται: ἐστὶν bO ‖ 26 ante πλέον add. φίλος O ‖ 27 ἔρρωσθε om. ac

12-17. Mss. MUVbO(=acd) 28 Ἱπποκράτης om. O ‖ 29 ἀναδόντες Ob^2 ‖ 30 ἀνέδοσαν O τε: δὲ O καὶ[1] om. bO post ξενίην add. τε b ὑπισχνεομένους ἔο V even by a suspicion.

But neither god nor Nature would promise me silver for coming, whence do not you, men of Abdera, force it on me, but leave free the work of a free science. People who put their knowledge out for hire require it to be slavish, exchanging its earlier freedom of speech for fetters. After that in all likelihood they may lie about a disease as though it were serious, and make disclaimers as though it were insignificant. They may not come when they have promised, and again may come uncalled. Man's life is a pitiful thing: through the whole of it, like a winter wind, has penetrated the unbearable love of money. If only all physicians would come together to cure a sickness which is worse than madness, because it is considered blessed, though it is a disease, and a ruinous one. In my view all affections of the soul are insanities which imprint certain extreme beliefs and fantasies on the reasoning faculty, and the man who is purged of them by means of virtue becomes sound. If I wanted to enrich myself by every means, oh Abderites, not for ten talents would I be coming to you. I would be going to the great king of the Persians where I would be given whole cities brimming with the good fortune that comes from men. I would be healing the plague there. But I refused to free a land inimical to Greece from the evil disease, I, too, fighting my naval battle against the barbarian in the way available to me. I would have acquired disgrace by acquiring wealth from the king and opulence inimical to my fatherland, and in wearing them I would exhibit my office as a destroyer of Greek cities.[1] Wealth comes not from moneymaking by any and all means. Great are virtue's sacred shrines to justice. They are not buried, but manifest. Or do you not think that it is an equal sin to save the enemy and to save friends for pay? That is not my way, oh people. I get no harvest from disease, nor was any prayer of mine answered when I heard of Democritus' derangement. He, if he is well, will be my friend, and if he is sick will be the more so when he is cured. My information is that he is a weighty man, solid of character and your city's jewel. Be well!

12. Hippocrates to Philopoimen. Greetings.

The ambassadors who delivered your city's letter also gave me yours. I was delighted at your promise to receive me and to offer other entertainment.

[1] ἑλέπολις is an Aeschylean word, from *Agamemnon* 689.

διαίτην. ἔλθοιμεν δ' ἂν αἰσίᾳ τύχῃ, καὶ ἀφιξόμεθα, ὡς ὑπολαμβάνομεν, χρηστοτέρῃσιν ἐλπίσιν, ὡς ἐν τῇ γραφῇ παραδεδήλωται, οὐ μανίην ἀλλὰ ψυχῆς τινα ῥῶσιν ὑπερβάλλουσαν διασαφηνέοντος τοῦ ἀνδρός, μήτε παίδων μήτε γυναικὸς μήτε ξυγγενέων μήτε οὐσίης μήτε τινὸς ὅλως ἐν φροντίδι ἐόντος, ἡμέρην δὲ καὶ εὐφρόνην πρὸς ἑωυτὸν καθεστεῶτος καὶ ἰδιάζοντος τὰ μὲν πολλὰ ἐν ἄντροισι καὶ ἠρεμίῃσι ὑπὸ σκιάσεσι δενδρέων ἢ ἐν μαλακῇσι ποίῃσιν ἢ παρ' ἡσύχοισιν ὑδάτων ῥείθροισι. συμβαίνει μὲν οὖν τὰ πολλὰ τοῖσι μελαγχολικοῖσι τοιαῦτα· σίγηροί τε γὰρ ἐνίοτέ εἰσιν καὶ μονήρεις καὶ φιλέρημοι τυγχάνουσι· ἀπανθρωπέονταί τε ξύμφυλον ὄψιν ἀλλοτρίην νομίζοντες. οὐκ ἀπεοικὸς δὲ καὶ τοῖσι περὶ παιδείην ἐσπουδακόσι τὰς ἄλλας φροντίδας ὑπὸ μιῆς τῆς ἐν σοφίῃ διαθέσεως σεσοβῆσθαι. ὥσπερ γὰρ δμῶές τε καὶ δμωΐδες ἐν τῇσιν οἰκίῃσιν θορυβέοντες καὶ στασιάζοντες, ὁκόταν ἐξαπιναίως αὐτοῖσιν ἡ δέσποινα ἐπιστῇ, πτοηθέντες ἀφησυχάζουσι, παραπλησίως καὶ αἱ λοιπαὶ κατὰ ψυχὴν ἐπιθυμίαι, ἀνθρώποισι κακῶν ὑπηρέτιδες· ἐπὴν δ' ἡ σοφίης ὄψις ἑωυτὴν ἐπιστήσῃ, ὡς δοῦλα τὰ λοιπὰ πάθεα ἐκκεχώρηκε. ποθέουσι δ'
332 ἄντρα καὶ ἡσυχίην οὐ πάν|τως οἱ μανέντες, ἀλλὰ καὶ οἱ τῶν ἀνθρωπίνων πρηγμάτων ὑπερφρονήσαντες ἀταραξίης ἐπιθυμίῃ. ὁκόταν γὰρ ὁ νοῦς ὑπὸ τῶν ἔξω θορύβων κοπτόμενος ἀναπαύσασθαι θελήσῃ, τὸ σῶμα τότε ταχέως ἐς ἡσυχίην μετήλλαξεν. εἶτα ἀναστὰς ὄρθιος ἐν ἑωυτῷ περιεσκόπει κύκλῳ χωρίον ἀληθείης, ἐν ᾧ οὐ πατήρ, οὐ γυνή, οὐ τέκνα, οὐ μήτηρ, οὐ κασίγνητος, οὐ ξυγγενεῖς, οὐ δμῶες, οὐ τύχη, οὐχ ὅλως οὐδὲν τῶν θόρυβον ἐμποιησόντων. πάντα δ' ἀποκεκλεισμένα τὰ ταράσσοντα ἕστηκεν ὑπὸ φόβου οὐδὲ πλησιάσαι τολμέοντα ὑπ' εὐλαβείης τῶν αὐτόθι οἰκεόντων. οἰκέουσι δὲ τὸ χωρίον ἐκεῖνο τέχναι καὶ ἀρεταὶ παντοῖαι καὶ θεοὶ καὶ δαίμονες καὶ βουλαὶ καὶ γνῶμαι, καὶ ὁ μέγας πόλος ἐν ἐκείνῳ τῷ χωρίῳ τοὺς πολυκινήτους ἀστέρας κατέστεπται, ἐς ὃ τάχα καὶ Δημόκριτος ὑπὸ σοφίης μετῴκισται. εἶτ' οὐκέτι ὁρέων τοὺς ἐν τῇ πόλει ἅτε τηλοῦ ἐκδεδημηκὼς δοξάζεται μανίης νοῦσον διὰ τὸ φιλέρημον. σπεύδουσι δὲ Ἀβδηρῖται ἀργυρίου ἐλεγχθῆναι, ὅτι οὐ ξυνιᾶσι Δημόκριτον. ἀλλὰ σύ γε ἡμῖν κατάρτυε τὴν ξεινίην, ὦ ἑταῖρε Φιλοποίμην. οὐ γὰρ ἐθέλω τεταραγμένῃ τῇ πόλει παρασχεῖν ὄχλησιν ἐκ παλαιοῦ ἴδιον ἔχων ξεῖνόν σε, ὡς οἶσθα. ἔρρωσο.

---

1 ἂν om. O ‖ 3 τοῦ om. O ‖ 5 ἱμέρην O δὲ: τε U εὐφροσύνην O εὐφρονέην V ἑωυτῷ MU ἑωϋτὸ V ἑωυτὸν b καθεστῶτα (-έωτα M)MVb ‖ 6 ἰδιάζοντα MVb τὰ μὲν πολλά: πάμπολλα O ἐρημίῃσιν b post ἠρεμ. add. ἢ O, ἢ ἐν b ὑπὸ σκιάσεσι: Putz. ὑποσκιάσεσι MUVb ὑπὸ σκέπεσι O ‖ 7 ἐν: καὶ O μαλθακέσι MUV πόαις MU παρὰ συχνοῖσι U παρησυχνοῖσι M ‖ 8 μελαγχολῶσι Ob[2] εἰσιν ἐνίοτε Vb εἰσιν om. O ‖ 9 ξύμφυλλον V ‖ 10 ἀλλοτριωτάτην O ‖ 12 σεσωβῆσθαι M τε: δὲ O om. b τε καὶ δμωΐδες om. V τοῖσιν οἴκοισι O ‖ 14 ἐφησυχάζουσι O ante καὶ add. δὲ U ante κατὰ add. αἱ O ‖ 15 δ' ἡ: δὲ MUO δὴ b ‖ 16 κεχώρηκε V δ' om. MU ‖ 17 οὐ πάντως οἱ: οὐ πάντες οὐ a ‖ 19 θορύβων: φροντίδων O σῶμα: στόμα V ‖ 20 ὄρθριος O ‖ 21 περισκοπεῖ bO οὐ πατήρ om. O ‖ 22 κασίγνητοι Ob[2] οὐ τύχη om. O οὐχ: οὐδ' O οὐθ' Vb οὐδὲν: οὐδὲ ἓν b τῶν: τὸν U ‖ 23 ἐμποιησάντων MU ἐμποιούντων O τὰ παράσσον (sic) U ‖ 25 ἐνοικεόντων b παντοῖαι om. O ‖ 28 μετοικήσας O ἅτε: οἷά γε O ‖ 30 ἐξελεγχθῆναι b ‖ 31 ὦ om. O οὐ: οὐδὲ bO ‖ 32 ξένον corr. in φίλον b ‖ 33 post οἶσθα add. σύ b ἔρρωσο om. O

Then we may come with good omens, and we shall come, as we suspect, with better hopes, as my letter showed, if the man is revealing not madness but an overwhelming strength of soul, having not children nor wife nor relatives nor property, nor anything at all on his mind, but day and night staying by himself and being mostly alone in caves and the quiet covering of trees or in soft grass, or by quiet streams of water. Such things are generally characteristic of melancholics. Sometimes they are quiet, solitary, and like deserted places. And they avoid people, considering the face of their own tribe alien. But it is not unlikely that when people are serious about learning, other concerns are put to flight by that one orientation to wisdom. Just as slaves, serving men and women who are making a tumult and quarreling in a house, when the mistress suddenly appears, cringe and fall silent, similarly the other passions of the soul, the ministers of men's wickedness; when the face of learning exhibits herself, all other affections, because they are slavish, withdraw. It is not wholly madmen who want caves and quiet, but also those who scorn human affairs in their desire for freedom from perturbation.[1] When the intellect wants to stop being battered by external tumult it takes the body quickly then to quiet. Then it stands upright in itself and looks round in a circle at the place of truth, where there is no father, no wife, children, mother, sibling, relatives, menials, no Chance, in sum, none of the things that will make a tumult. All things that perturb stay shut out by fear; out of respect for those who live there they dare not approach. And those who live in that place are the sciences, virtues of all sorts, the gods and demigods, will and thought. In that place the great pole has made a wreath of his restless stars. And there, perhaps, Democritus, too, has been removed by learning. And so, since he no longer sees those in the city because he has traveled so far, he is judged mad for his love of solitude. The Abderites want it proved, and will pay for it, that they don't understand Democritus. But do prepare to receive me, my dear Philopoimen. I am not willing to make trouble in a city so perturbed, and I have, as you know, an ancient relation of guest friendship with you. Be well!

---

[1] Ataraxia, the code word for the Epicureans for what they sought in retirement from the world.

13. Ἱπποκράτης Διονυσίῳ χαίρειν·

Ἢ περίμεινόν με ἐν Ἁλικαρνησσῷ ἢ φθάσον αὐτὸς ἐλθεῖν, ὦ ἑταῖρε.
334 κατὰ πᾶσαν γὰρ ἀνάγκην ἀπιτέον ἐς Ἄβδηρά μοι Δημο|κρίτεω χάριν, ἐφ' ὃν νοσέοντα μετεπέμψατό με ἡ πόλις. ἀλεκτός τις ἡ συμπαθείη τῶν ἀνθρώπων, Διονύσιε. ὡς μία ψυχὴ ξυννοσεῖ τῷ πολίτῃ, ὥστε μοι δοκέουσι καὶ αὐτοὶ θεραπείης δεῖσθαι. ἐγὼ δὲ οἶμαι οὐδὲ νοῦσον αὐτὸ εἶναι, ἀλλ' ἀμετρίην παιδείης, οὐκ οὖσάν γε τῷ ἔοντι ἀμετρίην, ἀλλὰ νομιζομένην τοῖσιν ἰδιώτῃσιν, ἐπεὶ οὐδέποτε βλαβερὸν τὸ ἀρετῆς ἄμετρον. δόξα δὲ νούσου γίνεται τοῦτο διὰ τὴν τῶν κρινόντων ἀπαιδευσίην· δοκιμάζει δ' ἕκαστος, ἐξ ὧν αὐτὸς οὐκ ἔχει, τὸ ἐν ἄλλῳ πλεονάζον περισσεύειν. ὥς που καὶ ὁ δειλὸς ἀμετρίην τὴν ἀνδρείην ὑπείληφε καὶ ὁ φιλάργυρος τὴν μεγαλοψυχίην, καὶ πᾶσα ἔλλειψις ὑπερβάλλειν δοκεῖ τὸ ἀρετῆς ξύμμετρον. ἐκεῖνον μὲν οὖν αὐτὸν ἰδόντες, μετὰ τῆς ἔνθεν δὲ προγνώσιος, καὶ ἀκούσαντες τῶν λόγων αὐτοῦ ἄμεινον εἰσόμεθα· σὺ δὲ ἔπειξον, ὦ Διονύσιε, αὐτὸς παραγενέσθαι. βούλομαι γὰρ ἐνδιατρῖψαί σε τῇ πατρίδι μου, μέχρις ἐπανέλθω, ὅκως τῶν τε ἡμετέρων φροντίζῃς καὶ πρὸ τῶν ἐμῶν τῆς πόλιος. ἐπειδὴ οὐκ οἶδ' ὅκως ἐκ συντυχίης ὑγιεινὸν τὸ ἔτος ἐστὶ καὶ τὴν ἀρχαίην φύσιν ἔχον, ὥστε οὐ πολλαὶ παρενοχλήσουσι νοῦσοι. πλὴν ὅμως πάριθι. οἰκήσεις δὲ τὴν ἐμὴν οἰκίην ὑπερευκαιρέουσαν, ἅτε καὶ τοῦ γυναίου μένοντος πρὸς τοὺς γονέας διὰ τὴν ἐμὴν ἐκδημίην. ἐπισκόπει δὲ ὅμως καὶ τὰ ἐκείνης ὅκως διάγῃ σωφρόνως καὶ μὴ τὴν ἀνδρὸς ἀπουσίην ἄλλους ἄνδρας νομίσῃ. κόσμιον μὲν γὰρ ἐξ ἀρχῆς ἦν καὶ γονέας ἀστείους εἶχε, τὸν δὲ πατέρα ἐκτόπως ἀνδρικόν τε καὶ μάλα μισοπόνηρον |
336 ὑπερφυῶς γερόντιον. ἀλλ' ὅμως ἀεὶ χρῄζει γυνὴ σωφρονίζοντος· ἔχει γὰρ φύσει τὸ ἀκόλαστον ἐν ἑωυτῇ, ὅπερ, εἰ μὴ καθ' ἡμέρην ἐπικόπτοιτο, ὡς τὰ δένδρα καθυλομανεῖ. ἐγὼ δὲ φίλον οἴομαι ἀκριβέστερον γονέων ἐς φυλακὴν γυναικός· οὐ γὰρ ὡς ἐκείνοισι καὶ τούτῳ ξυνοικεῖ πόθος εὐνοίης, δι' οὗ πολλάκις ἐπισκιάζεται τὴν νουθεσίην. φρονιμώτερον δὲ ἐν παντὶ τὸ ἀπαθέστερον ἅτε μὴ ἐπικλώμενον ὑπ' εὐνοίης. ἔρρωσο.

---

1 Ἱπποκ. et χαίρειν om. O ‖ 2 ἁλικαρνασῷ O ἐλθὼν O ‖ 3 Ἄβδηράν MU ‖ 4 ἀλεκτός τις b ἀλλ' ἐκτός τις V ἄλεκτος γάρ τις O ἀλλ' ἐκτοπός τις MU ‖ 5-6 ὥς τέ μοι δοκέει θεραπείης δέεσθαι καὶ αὐτοὶ V ‖ 6 δὲ: μὲν O νοῦσου O αὐτὸ: αὐτὴν corr. in αὐτῷ M αὐτῷ U ‖ 7 γε: δὲ O ‖ 9 τοῦτο: τὸ ὑπερβάλλον MUVb ‖ 10 ὥς: καὶ ἴσως O ‖ 13 ἔνθεν δὲ scripsi ἐνθένδε mss. ‖ 15 αὐτὸς om. O ‖ 16 τε om. Vb φροντιεῖς MUVb ἡμῶν corr. in ἐμῶν M ‖ 17 ἐπεὶ Vb ἐπεὶ δὲ U ἔπειτ' O ‖ 18 οὐδὲ MUV πολλὰ O νοῦσοι: σοι MU ‖ 19 τὴν ἐμὴν εὐκαιροῦσαν οἰκ. O ‖ 20 ἀποδημίην O ‖ 21 ὅμως om. O τὰ: τὰς a ‖ 21 post μὴ add. διὰ O post τὴν add. τοῦ O τῇ...ἀπουσίῃ b (corr. b^2) ‖ 22 γὰρ: οὖν O ἦν om. O ante γον. add. τοὺς O ‖ 23 ἐκτόκως V ἐκτόπως om. O μάλα om. O ‖ 24 χρῄζει: δεῖται U ante γυνὴ add. ἡ U ante σωφρον.add. τοῦ b ‖ 25 φύσῃ V ante τὸ add. καὶ VbO μὴ om. U^2 (U hic illegibilis) μὴ post ἡμέρην O ἐκκόπτοιτο ὥσπερ O ‖ 26 ἀκριβέστερον οἶμαι O post ἀκριβ. add. οἶδα b^2 ‖ 27 τούτῳ: τουτέοισι O πάθος bO ‖ 28 δι' οὗ: διὸ O ἐπισκιάζονται O ‖ 29 ἅτε μή: ἐὰν ᾖ O ὑπ': ἐπ' U ἔρρωσο om. O

13. Hippocrates to Dionysius. Greetings.

Either wait for me in Halicarnassus or hurry to come, my friend. It is entirely necessary for me to go to Abdera for the sake of Democritus, to whom the city has summoned me because he is sick. The sympathy of the people is indescribable, Dionysius. Like a single soul the city has fallen ill with its citizen. Hence they, themselves, seem to me to need treatment. And I think that his is not even an illness, but an excess of learning. No, not truly an excess, though it is thought so by laymen, since excess of excellence is never harmful. The judgment of sickness comes from the ignorance of those judging. Every man makes an assessment in accord with his own deficiency, that what someone else has more of he considers excessive. Thus the coward supposes that courage, and the greedy man that generosity, is excess. Every deficiency thinks reasonable virtue is excessive. When I have seen the man in person, and after a prognosis on the spot, and after I have heard him talk I shall know better.

But do you hurry to join me, Dionysius. I want you to stay in my homeland until I come back, so that you can take care of my affairs and even before mine, those of the city. For somehow by luck it is a healthy year with its primal nature,[1] so that few diseases will come to make trouble. Still, come anyway. You will live in my house, which will be very convenient since my dear little wife will stay with her parents because of my absence. But still, look after her affairs, so that she behaves in a disciplined way and doesn't think that a husband's absence means other men. She has been proper from the first; she had very civilized parents, an extremely manly father: a dear old fellow who hates rascals. But a woman always needs someone to discipline her. By nature she has the untamable in her and unless it is pruned day by day it goes wild, like trees.[2] And I think a friend is more punctilious than parents in guarding a wife. He, unlike them, does not have an indwelling desire for amity, on account of which one often puts correction in the shade. Lack of emotion is wisest in all things since it is not deflected by amity. Be well!

---

[1] ἀρχαίη φύσις is a fairly common phrase in the Hippocratic writings for the original state of an organ or bodily member which therapy seeks to restore (see, e.g., *Epid.* 2.2.6, 2.8.4), but it is not used, as it apparently is here, for the natural constitution of the year with heat, cold, wet, and dry at the proper times. (cf. *Airs Waters Places* ch. 10)

[2] ὑλομανεῖ, in botanical terms, "going crazy for wood," occurs in plants because of excess nutrition. E.g., Theophrastus, *De causis plantarum* 3.1.5, ἄκαρπος γίνεται καθάπερ ὑλομανῶν καὶ ἐξυβρίζων. Cutting it back restrains its hybris and makes it more productive of fruit. See Ann Michelini, "'ΥΒΡΙΣ and Plants," *HSCP* 82 (1978) 35-44, who quotes the example from Theophrastus.

14. Ἱπποκράτης Δαμαγήτῳ χαίρειν·

Οἶδα παρὰ σοὶ γενόμενος ἐν Ῥόδῳ, Δαμάγητε, τὴν ναῦν ἐκείνην, Ἅλιος ἐπιγραφὴ ἦν αὐτῇ, πάγκαλόν τινα καὶ εὔπρυμνον ἱκανῶς ⟨τε⟩ τετροπισμένην, καὶ διάβασιν εἶχε πολλήν. ἐπῄνεις δὲ καὶ τὸ ναυτικὸν αὐτῆς ὡς ὀξὺ καὶ ἀσφαλὲς καὶ εὔτεχνον ὑπουργῆσαι καὶ τοῦ πλοῦ τὴν εὐδρομίην. ταύτην ἔκπεμψον ἡμῖν, ἀλλ' εἰ οἷόν τε μὴ κώπησιν, ἀλλὰ πτεροῖσιν ἐρετμώσας αὐτήν. ἐπείγει γὰρ τὸ πρῆγμα, φιλότης, καὶ μάλα ἐς Ἄβδηρα διαπλεῦσαι πάνυ ταχέως. βούλομαι γὰρ νοσέουσαν ἰήσασθαι πόλιν διὰ νοσέοντα ἕνα Δημόκριτον. ἀκούεις που τἀνδρὸς τὸ κλέος· τοῦτον ἡ πατρὶς ᾐτίηται μανίῃ κεκακῶσθαι· ἐγὼ δὲ βούλομαι, μᾶλλον δὲ εὔχομαι μὴ ἐόντως αὐτὸν παρακόπτειν, ἀλλ' ἐκείνοισιν δόξαν εἶναι.
338 γελᾷ, φασίν, αἰεὶ καὶ οὐ παύεται γε|λῶν ἐπὶ παντὶ πρήγματι καὶ σημεῖον αὐτοῖσι μανίης τοῦτο δοκεῖ. ὅθεν λέγε τοῖσιν ἐν Ῥόδῳ φίλοισι μετριάζειν ἀεὶ καὶ μὴ πολλὰ γελᾶν μηδὲ πολλὰ σκυθρωπάζειν, ἀλλὰ τούτων ἀμφοῖν τὸ μέτριον κτήσασθαι, ἵνα τοῖσι μὲν χαριέστατος εἶναι δόξῃς, τοῖσι δὲ φροντιστὴς περὶ ἀρετὴν μερμηρίζων. ἔνι μέντοι τι, Δαμάγητε, κακὸν παρ' ἕκαστον αὐτοῦ γελῶντος. εἰ γὰρ ἡ ἀμετρίη φλαῦρον, τὸ διὰ παντὸς φλαυρότερον. καὶ εἴποιμ' ἂν αὐτῷ· Δημόκριτε, καὶ νοσέοντος καὶ κτεινομένου καὶ τεθνεῶτος καὶ πολιορκουμένου καὶ παντὸς ἐμπίπτοντος κακοῦ ἕκαστον τῶν πρησσομένων ὕλη σοι γέλωτος ὑπόκειται. οὐ θεομαχεῖς δέ, εἰ δύο ἐόντων ἐν κόσμῳ, λύπης καὶ χαρᾶς, σὺ θάτερον αὐτῶν ἐκβέβληκας; μακάριός τ' ἂν ἦς, ἀλλ' ἀδύνατον, εἰ μήτε μήτηρ σοι νενόσηκε μήτε πατὴρ μήτε τὰ ὕστερον τέκνα ἢ γυνὴ ἢ φίλος, ἀλλὰ διὰ τὸν σὸν γέλωτα, ἵνα σῴζηται, εὐτυχεῖς πάντα. ἀλλὰ νοσεόντων γελᾷς, ἀποθνῃσκόντων χαίρεις, εἴ τι που πύθοιο κακόν, εὐφραίνει· ὡς πονηρότατος εἶ, ὦ Δημόκριτε, καὶ πόρρω γε σοφίης. ἢ νομίζεις αὐτὰ μηδὲ κακὰ εἶναι; μελαγχολᾷς οὖν, Δημόκριτε, κινδυνεύων καὶ αὐτὸς Ἀβδηρίτης εἶναι, φρονιμωτέρη δὲ ἡ πόλις. ἀλλὰ περὶ μὲν δὴ τούτων ἀκριβέστερον ἐκεῖσε λέξομεν, Δαμάγητε. ἡ δὲ ναῦς καὶ τὸν χρόνον, ὃν ἐπιστέλλω σοι, χρονίζει. ἔρρωσο.

---

1 Ἱππoκ. om. O || 2 ante Ἅλιος add. ἣ b || 3 τε: add. Corn. || 4 πολλήν om. U || 5 ἔντεχνον O || 6 ἀλλ' om. O || 7 αὐτήν om. Vb γὰρ: οὖν O || 8 γὰρ om. bO || 9 τὸ κλέος τοῦ ἀνδρός O || 10 αἰτιῆται O ἡγεῖται conj. b^2 δὲ[I] : τε O δὲ[II] : καὶ U || 11 δόξας V δόξαν corr. in δόξας M δόξα γίνεται (om. εἶναι) O || 12 γελᾶν U φησὶν O οὐδέποτε O καὶ[II] om. O || 13 αὐτοῖσι: αὐτὸ O αὐτῆς U τοῦτο μανίης bO in marg. ante ὅθεν add. τοῦτο δὲ καὶ ἔσωθεν b^2 || 13-14 αἰεὶ μετρ. b ||14 ἀεὶ om. VO post σκυθρωπ. add. ἀεὶ U ἀλλὰ: καὶ ἄλλα U || 15 κυήσασθαι VMm (corr. M^2) κτίσασθαι U post κτ. add. παρὰ Ἀβδηριτῶν b δόξῃς scripsi δόξειας mss. τοῖσι[II]: οἷς mss. corr. Corn. || 16 ἀρετῆς bO ἕν εἴ τι μέντοι τι M ἔνι: ἐνὶ V τι om. O || 17 διὰ παντὸς: διαπαν U || 18 καὶ[1] om. V || 19 κρινομένου b^2 κτιννυμένου O || 21 ἐόντοιν O || 22 αὐτῶν om. O τ' om. V μήτε om. V ἡ μήτηρ O || 23 ἢ…ἢ: μὴ…μὴ O ἀλλὰ: ἀλλ' εἰ U || 24 ἵνα σῴζηται: ἵνα διασώζηται M πάντα σώζεται U τὰ post εὐτυχεῖς add. O ἀλλὰ: τὰ ἄλλα MV || 25 ante χαίρεις add. δὲ U || 26 ὦ om. O ἦ b ἣν νομίζῃς U || 27 ante Δημ. add. ὦ O κινδυνεύω O || 28 φρονιμώτερος b (corr b^2) ἡ om. O δὴ om. UVO ἐκεῖ O || 29 λέξωμεν U post χρόνον add. τοῦτον UbO ante ὃν add καθ' U ὧν M || 30 ἔρρωσο om. O

14. Hippocrates to Damagetus. Greetings.

Having been with you in Rhodes, Damagetus, I know that fine vessel, Helios she was called,[1] with the fine stern, a sturdy keel and and good deck space. You praised her seaworthiness too, said she was lively, safe, and precise to handle, and swift of passage. Send her to us, fitting her if you can, with wings for oars.[2] The business is pressing, dear friend; indeed I must sail to Abdera with all speed. I want to cure a city which is sick because of the sickness of a single man, Democritus. You have heard of his reputation, no doubt. His city has accused him of being undone by madness. It is my wish, rather my prayer, that he is not truly mad but seems so to them. He laughs continually, they say, and never stops. He laughs at everything, and that seems a sign of madness to them. So tell your friends at Rhodes to be ever moderate, never laugh much nor be stern much, but acquire moderation in both, so that you will seem very charming to some people, and to others a deep thinker meditating on virtue. But there is something bad in his laughing at everything, Damagetus. If excess is wicked, then unremitting excess is more so. I may say to him, "Democritus, when people are sick, being killed, dead, besieged, subject to any evil, everything that happens to them is matter for laughter to you. Are you not fighting the gods when, since the universe holds grief and joy, two things, you have rejected one? You would be blessed (But this cannot happen!) if your mother never fell ill, nor your father, nor again your children, nor your wife or friend, but, for the sake of your laughter, so that it could be maintained, they were fortunate in all respects. But people do get ill, and you laugh. They do die and you are delighted. If you should learn of something bad, you become cheerful. What a vile fellow you are, Democritus, and how far from wisdom. Or do you think these things are not evils? You are melancholic, then, Democritus, in danger of being a proper Abderite, and the city is wiser than you." But we shall speak more in detail about these things there, Damagetus. Your ship is wasting time even while I am writing to you. Be well!

---

[1] Lionel Casson, *Ships and Seamanship in the Ancient World* (Princeton: 1971) 346 n. 7, would translate "Halios was the painted device on it." Rhodes had an active cult of the god Helios, in honor of whom the Halieia was celebrated. (See H. J. Rose, *OCD*, s.v. Helios, for bibliography.) Casson says that this is the earliest instance of a name of a merchant ship that we know, but he is probably assuming too early a date for this letter.

[2] Alluding probably to Aeschylus, *Agamemnon* 52, πτερύγων ἐρετμοῖσιν ἐρεσσόμενοι, the eagles "rowing with wings for oars."

15. Ἱπποκράτης Φιλοποίμενι χαίρειν·

Σύννους καὶ πεφροντικὼς ὑπὲρ Δημοκρίτεω αὐτῇ ἐκείνῃ τῇ νυκτὶ καταδαρθὼν πρὸς ἀρχομένην τὴν ἕω ὄναρ ἐφαντάσθην, ἐξ οὗ νομίζω
340 κάρτα μηδὲν ἐπισφαλὲς γενήσεσθαι· ἐκπάγλως δὲ διηγέρθην. | ἐδόκεον γὰρ αὐτὸν τὸν Ἀσκληπιὸν ὁρᾶν· φαίνεσθαί τε αὐτὸν πλησίον· ἤδη δὲ πρὸς τῇσιν τῶν Ἀβδηριτῶν πύλῃσιν ἐτυγχάνομεν. ὁ δὲ Ἀσκληπιὸς οὐχ ὡς εἰώθεσαν αὐτοῦ αἱ εἰκόνες μείλιχός τε καὶ πρᾶος ἰδέσθαι κατεφαίνετο, ἀλλὰ διεγηγερμένος τῇ σχέσει καὶ ἰδέσθαι φοβερώτερος. εἵποντο δὲ αὐτῷ δράκοντες σχήματι ἑρπετῶν ὑπερφυεῖς, ἐπειγόμενοι δὲ καὶ αὐτοὶ μακρῷ τῷ ἐπισύρματι καί τι φρικῶδες ὡς ἐν ἐρημίῃ καὶ νάπῃσι κοίλῃσι ὑποσυρίζοντες. οἱ δὲ κατόπιν ἑταῖροι κίστας φαρμάκων εὖ μάλα περιεσφηκωμένας ἔχοντες ᾔεσαν. ἔπειτα ὤρεξέ μοι τὴν χεῖρα ὁ θεὸς κἀγὼ λαβόμενος ἀσμένως ἐλιπάρεον ξυνέρχεσθαι καὶ μὴ καθυστερεῖν μου τῆς θεραπείης. ὁ δέ· Οὐδέν τι, ἔφη, ἐν τῷ παρεόντι ἐμεῦ χρήζεις, ἀλλά σε αὕτη τὰ νῦν ξεναγήσει θεὸς κοινὴ ἀθανάτων τε καὶ θνητῶν. ἐγὼ δὲ ἐπιστραφεὶς ὁρέω γυναῖκα καλήν τε καὶ μεγάλην, ἀφελὲς πεπλοκισμένην, λαμπρείμονα. διέλαμπον δ' αὐτῆς οἱ τῶν ὀμμάτων κύκλοι καθαρόν τι φῶς, οἷον ἀστέρων μαρμαρυγὰς δοκεῖν. καὶ ὁ μὲν δαίμων ἐχωρίσθη, κείνη δὲ ἡ γυνὴ πιέσασά με τοῦ καρποῦ μαλακῇ τινι εὐτονίῃ διὰ τοῦ ἄστεος ἦγε φιλοφρονεομένη. ὡς δὲ πλησίον τῆς οἰκίης ἦμεν ἵνα τὴν ξεινίην ἐδόκεον εὐτρεπίσθαι, ἀπῄει ὡς φάσμα μόνον εἰποῦσα· αὔριόν σε παρὰ Δημοκρίτεῳ καταλήψομαι. ἤδη δὲ αὐτῆς μεταστρεφομένης· Δέομαι, φημί, ἀρίστη, τίς εἶ καὶ τίνα σε καλέομεν; ἡ δέ· Ἀλήθεια,
342 ἔφη, αὕτη δέ, ἣν προσιοῦσαν ὁρῇς, καὶ | ἐξαίφνης ἑτέρη τις κατεφαίνετό μοι οὐκ ἀκαλλὴς μὲν οὐδ' αὐτή, θρασυτέρη δὲ ἰδέσθαι καὶ σεσοβημένη, Δόξα, ἔφη, καλεῖται. κατοικεῖ δὲ παρὰ τοῖσιν Ἀβδηρίτῃσιν. ἐγὼ μὲν οὖν ἀναστὰς ὑπεκρινάμην ἐμαυτῷ τοὖναρ, ὅτι οὐ δέοιτο ἰητροῦ Δημόκριτος, ὅπου γε αὐτὸς ὁ θεραπεύων θεὸς ἀπέστη ὡς οὐκ ἔχων ὕλην θεραπείης. ἀλλὰ ἡ μὲν Ἀλήθεια τοῦ ὑγιαίνειν παρὰ Δημοκρίτεῳ μένει, ἡ δὲ τοῦ νοσεῖν αὐτὸν Δόξα παρὰ Ἀβδηρίτῃσιν ἐόντως κατῴκηκε. ταῦτα πιστεύω ἀληθέα εἶναι, Φιλοποίμην, καὶ ἐστί. οὐκ ἀπογινώσκω τὰ ὀνείρατα,

---

1 Ἱπποκρ. om. O ‖ 2 αὐτῇ om. O ‖ 3 καταδαρθῶν MUV -άρθων b ἀρχομένῃ τῇ O ἠῶ V ἠῷ b (corr. b²) ὄνειρα τί U ἐφαντάσθη V ‖ 4 γεγενῆσθαι O ἐκπάγλως: ἐκπλαγὸς V ἔκπλακτος b ἔκπαλτός O δὲ: τε UO γὰρ δὲ M ἐδοκέω U ‖ 5 τε om. MV αὐτῷ b αὐτοῦ UV αὐτέου M δὲ: καὶ U ‖ 6 τῶν: αὐτῶν U om. bO ‖ 7 μείλιχόν τε (τι b) καὶ πρᾶον MVb μέλιχρόν τι b² ‖ 8 διεγειγερμένος MU ‖ 9 ἐν σχήματι ἑρπετῷ U χρῆμά τι bO ὑπερφυὲς O καὶ om. U αὐτῷ U ‖ 10 ἐρημίῃσι U ‖ 11 ἕτεροι V ἑτέροι MU ‖ 12 εἶτα U om. ἔπειτα, add. δὲ post ὤρεξε O ‖ 13 ἄσμενος O ἐσσυμένως b (corr. b²) μου: μοι MU τι μου O ‖ 14 χρήζεις ἐμέο O ‖ 15 τὰ νῦν om. O τὰ νῦν αὕτη U ‖ 16 ἀσφαλὲς MO ἀσφαλῶς U ‖ 18 ἀμαρυγὰς b ‖ 19 πιέξασα O ‖ 21 εὐτρεπεῖσθαι M εὐτρεπιεῖσθαι b μόνον: οἷον b ‖ 23 ἔφην O ἀλήθειαν U ‖ 24 αὐτὴν M post καὶ add. γὰρ O μοι om. O ‖ 25 οὐ κακὴ O οὐκ ἄλλης M οὐ κακὸ U οὐδ': ἦδ' U ἰδέσθαι om. O ἰδέειν U ‖ 26 ante ἔφη add. δ' b τῇσιν V μὲν om. O ‖ 27 ὑπεκρινόμην V δεήσοιτο O ‖ 28 ὡς om. O ‖ 29-30 παρὰ…Δόξα om. U ‖ 30 κατοικέει O ‖ 31 ante Φιλοπ. add. ὦ b² ante οὐκ add. καὶ UbO

15. Hippocrates to Philopoimen. Greetings.

I was anxious, thinking about Democritus on this very night. Falling asleep towards the break of dawn I had a dream, after which I believe that nothing dangerous will happen. And I woke up in an amazing state. I seemed to see Asclepius himself, and he appeared to be near to me.[1] We were already near the gates of Abdera. Asclepius did not appear as his representations generally show him, sweet and gentle, but he was agitated in his bearing and rather frightening to look at. Snakes accompanied him, tremendous ones in the manner of crawling creatures, pressing on with great slithering, with terrifying hissing, as they do in deserted places and hollow valleys. Behind him his companions came with baskets of drugs tightly bound. The god stretched out his hand to me, and I took it and with joy begged him to come along and not desert me in the therapy. He said, "You have no need of me in the present case, but for now this common goddess of mortals and immortals will be your guide." I turned around and saw a large beautiful woman with her hair braided simply. She was radiant. The circles of her eyes showed forth a pure light. You would think it was the glistering of stars. The god withdrew and the woman took my wrist with a gentle pressure and led me through the town kindly. As we came near the house where they seemed to be preparing to entertain me she went off like a phantom, only saying "Tomorrow I shall find you at Democritus' house." And as she turned away I said, "I beg you, excellent one, who are you and what shall we call you?" "Truth," she said. "And this one you see approaching," and suddenly another woman appeared, not unhandsome herself, but bolder and agitated, "is named Opinion. She lives with the Abderites."[2]

I woke and analyzed my dream. It meant that Democritus does not need a physician, since the healing god stayed away because he had no grounds for giving treatment. But the Truth of his being healthy stays with Democritus and the Opinion that he is sick has truly made her home among Abderites. I believe

---

[1] Asclepius appears to his worshippers in dreams, at his shrines and elsewhere. Material is collected by Emma and Ludwig Edelstein, *Asclepius* (Baltimore: 1945). Hippocrates confidently interprets his dream himself, and needs no interpreter. Artemidorus, if consulted, would have told him that dreaming of Asclepius as a statue on his statue base is best. Dreaming of him in motion and going to a well person's house is a bad sign, while dreaming of him going to a sick person's house is good. (Artemidorus, *Onirocritica* 2.37, Pack p. 168.) Why is Asclepius agitated in Hippocrates' dream? Perhaps his loss of the placidity characteristic of his statues indicates his concern about Democritus. Dreaming of snakes is significant (Artem. *Onir*. 2.13, Pack 236-8), but the snakes of Hippocrates' dream are simply iconographical companions of Asclepius. Hippocrates' dream, which creates and interprets its own allegory, is more of a literary dream than are the dreams dealt with by Artemidorus or by the Hippocratic *Regimen* 4.

[2] The goddesses Truth and Opinion of Hippocrates' dream are reminiscent of the two figures in Prodicus' story of the choice of Heracles, as Xenophon tells it (*Mem*. 2.1.21-34). In Xenophon one of the two huge women, whose name turns out to be Virtue (Ἀρετή), is handsome and respectable (εὐπρεπῆ τε ἰδεῖν καὶ ἐλευθέριον φύσει) and modestly dressed, while the other, called Happiness (Εὐδαιμονία) by her friends, but Vice (Κακία) by her enemies, is soft and overfed (τεθραμμένην εἰς πολυσαρκίαν καὶ ἁπαλότητα), heavily made up and immodestly dressed.

μάλιστα δὲ ὁκόταν καὶ τάξιν διαφυλάττῃ. ἰητρικὴ δὲ καὶ μαντικὴ καὶ πάνυ ξυγγενεῖς εἰσίν, ἐπεὶ καὶ τῶν δυοῖν τεχνέων πατὴρ εἷς Ἀπόλλων, ὁ καὶ πρόγονος ἡμέων ἐούσας καὶ ἐσομένας νούσους προαγορεύων καὶ νοσέοντας καὶ νοσήσαντας ἰώμενος. ἔρρωσο.

16. Ἱπποκράτης Κρατεύᾳ χαίρειν·

Ἐπίσταμαί σε ῥιζοτόμον ἄριστον, ὦ ἑταῖρε, καὶ διὰ τὴν ἄσκησιν καὶ διὰ προγόνων κλέος, ὡς μηδὲν ἀποδεῖν σε τοῦ προπάτορος Κρατεύα. νῦν οὖν, εἰ καί ποτε ἄλλοτε, βοτανολόγησον, ὁκόσα τε καὶ ὁκοῖα δύνασαι, ἀναγκαίη γὰρ ἐπείγει, καὶ διάπεμψαί μοι ταῦτα ἐπ' ἄνδρα ὅλῃ πόλει ἰσοστάσιον, Ἀβδηρίτην μέν, ἀλλὰ Δημόκριτον. νοσεῖν γάρ φασιν αὐτὸν καὶ καθάρσιος μάλα χρῄζειν ἐντὸς μανίης ἐόντα. μὴ χρησαίμεθα μέντοι τοῖσι φαρμάκοισιν, ὥσπερ καὶ πέπεισμαι, ἀλλ' ὅμως εὐτρεπίσθαι χρὴ
344 πανταχόθεν. τὸ δὲ χρῆμα | τῶν βοτανῶν παρὰ σοὶ πολλάκις ἐθαύμασα καὶ τὴν τῶν ὅλων φύσιν τε καὶ διάταξιν καὶ τὸ ἱερώτατον γῆς ἵδρυμα, ἐξ ἧς ζῷα καὶ φυτὰ καὶ τροφαὶ καὶ φάρμακα καὶ τύχη καὶ ὁ πλοῦτος αὐτὸς ἀναφύεται. οὐδὲ γὰρ εἶχεν οἷ ἐπιβῇ ἡ φιλαργυρίη οὐδ' ἂν Ἀβδηρῖταί με νῦν δέκα ταλάντοισιν ἐδελέαζον, ἀντὶ ἰητροῦ μισθωτὸν ἐλέγχοντες. εἰ δ' ἐδύνασο, Κρατεύα, τῆς φιλαργυρίης τὴν πικρὰν ῥίζαν ἐκκόψαι, ὡς μηδὲν αὐτῆς λείψανον ἀφεῖναι, εὖ ἴσθι, ἐκαθήραμεν ἂν τῶν ἀνθρώπων μετὰ τῶν σωμάτων καὶ τὰς ψυχὰς νοσεούσας. ἀλλὰ ταῦτα μὲν εὐχαί· σὺ δ' ἡμῖν τὸ παρεὸν μάλιστα τὰς ὀρεινὰς καὶ ὑψηλολόφους βοτάνας ῥιζοτόμει· στερεώτεραι γὰρ τῶν ὑδρηλοτέρων εἰσὶν καὶ δριμύτεραι μᾶλλον διὰ τὴν τῆς γῆς πυκνότητα καὶ τὴν λεπτότητα τοῦ ἠέρος· ὅτι γὰρ ἕλκουσιν ἐμψυχρότερόν ἐστιν. πειρήθητι δ' ὅμως καὶ τὰς παρὰ λίμνῃσιν ἐλείους πεφυκυίας ἀνθολογῆσαι καὶ τὰς παραποταμίους ἢ κρηνίτιδας ἢ πιδακίτιδας παρ' ὑμῖν καλεομένας, ἃς ἀσθενέας καὶ ἀτόνους καὶ γλυκυχύλους εἶναι πέπεισμαι. πάντα δέ, ὁκόσα χυλοί τε καὶ ὀποὶ ῥέοντες, ἐν ὑαλίνοισιν ἀγγείοισι φερέσθωσαν, ὁκόσα δ' αὖ φύλλα ἢ ἄνθεα ἢ ῥίζαι, ἐν κώθωσι καινοῖσι περιεσφηκωμένοισιν, ὅκως μὴ διαυγαζόμενα τῇσι πνοῇσι ἐκλίπῃ τὸν τόνον τῆς φαρμακίης ὥσπερ ἀπολειποψυχήσαντα.

---

1 διαφυλάττοι O διαφυλάττει MU ‖ 1-2 πανὺ μαντιῇ συγγενής ἐστιν O ‖ 2 πάνυ: πάντῃ V ἐπειδὴ b καὶ om. O δύο M εἷς πατὴρ ὁ Ἀπόλλων O ‖ 3 ἡμῖν O ἐούσας καὶ om. O ἐσομένους U προαγορεύειν M ‖ 4 καὶ νοσήσαντας om. O ἔρρωσο om. O ‖ 5 Ἱπποκράτης om. O ‖ 6 ὦ om. bO ‖ 7 τὸ προγόνων O post σε add. δυνάμει b ‖ 8 οἷα UO ‖ 9 ἀναγκαίη γὰρ ἐπείγει: *Il.* 6.85, *Od.* 19.72 ταῦτα: αὐτὰ bO ‖ 10 αὐτόν φασι O ‖ 11 μέντοι: μὲν οὖν UO μὲν οὖν σου b[2] ‖ 12 εὐτρεπεῖσθαι M εὐτρεπιεῖσθαι b εὐτρεπίσασθαι O ‖ 13 πολλάκις παρά σοι O ‖ 14 ante καὶ[1] add. ὡς UbO ὅλων γε b ‖ 15 τὰ ζῷα καὶ τὰ φυτὰ O αὐτὸς om. U ‖ 16 ἂν εἶχε ποῖ ἐπιβῇ U ἡ om. M ‖ 17 εἰ δ': εἴθε δὲ O εἴθε δὲ εἰ b ‖ 19 ante ἐκαθήραμεν add. ὡς b ἐκάθηρες ἂν U ‖ 20 ψυχαῖς U νοσεούσας om. O ‖ 21 ὑψηλοφύτους O ὑψιλοφόρους U ὑψιλολόφους b ῥιζοτόμει βοτάνας O ‖ 22 γὰρ om. a ‖ 24 ἐμψυχότερον UbO λίμνας M ‖ 25 ποταμίους UVb κρηνήτιδας UVO ‖ 25-6 ἢ πιδακ. om. O ἢ πιδακ.... καλεομ. om. V ‖ 26 ἡμῖν O ἃς om. UMVO ‖ 27 τε om. O ‖ 28 ὑελίοισιν V ὑελίνοις U ὑαλίοισι M ὑελοῖς O αὖ: ἂν bO πάνθεα VM ‖ 29 ἢ ῥίζαι om. O καινοῖσι om. O διαυζόμενα M (corr. M[2]) διαρριπιζόμενα O ‖ 30 πνοιῇσιν bO ἐκλείπει M ἐκλείπῃ b ἐκλίπει U ἀποψυχήσαντα OM[2] λειποψυχήσαντα (λιπ. U) Ub

that this is true, Philopoimen, and it is. I do not deny dreams, especially when they retain coherence. Medicine and prophecy are very closely related, since of the two arts Apollo is the single father. He, who is my ancestor, declares the diseases that are and that will be and he heals those on whom sickness is coming and has come. Be well!

16. Hippocrates to Crateuas.[1] Greetings.

I know that you are an excellent herbalist, my friend, because of your training and your ancestors' fame, so that you are not inferior to the Crateuas who founded your family. Now, if ever, gather herbs, as many and as varied as you can, for necessity presses, and send them to me for a man equal in worth to a whole city–he is an Abderite, but he is Democritus. They say that he is sick and needs a purge because he is in the midst of madness. I hope we won't use the drugs. I believe we will not, but I must be ready for everything. The phenomenon of plants I have often admired in your company, and the nature and arrangement of the universe, and the holy foundation of the earth, whence animals, plants, food and drugs, luck and wealth itself springs forth. Without it, love of money would have no place to stand nor would the Abderites be tempting me with ten talents, accusing me of being a mercenary instead of a physician. If you, Crateuas, could cut the bitter root of love of money so as to leave nothing behind, know well we would purge the sick minds of men along with their bodies. But that is a prayer. For the present, gather especially the plants from mountains and high ridges. They are denser than the more moist ones and more bitter because of the thickness of the soil and the thinness of the air.[2] What they absorb is colder. But yet try to gather blossoms from marsh flowers by the ponds, river flowers, and fountain

---

[1] The famous Crateuas was physician to Mithridates VI Eupator, who died in 63 B.C., who concocted the antidote Mithridaticum. Crateuas was famous for his very popular, illustrated herbal, which was much used and referred to. Pliny, *N. H.* 25.8, says that it was alphabetic. In addition he wrote an alphabetic, scholarly description of plants, called the Ῥιζοτομικόν, much used by Dioscorides. I suspect that the audience was expected to think of that famous Crateuas and to think that Hippocrates is dealing with an ancestor of his. The title of Alexis' play, Κρατεύας ἢ Φαρμακοπώλης, suggests that the audience might well know of an earlier Crateuas (see above, the Introduction, n. 51). The ten fragments of Crateuas (from the margin of the sixth century Dioscorides manuscript, Vind. Med. 1) were published by Max Wellmann, *Krateuas. Abh. könig. Gesellschaft zu Göttingen*, Phil-hist. Kl., N. F. 3, Nr. 1 (Berlin: 1897), and with testimonia for Crateuas in his edition of Dioscorides, *Materia Medica* vol. III (Berlin: 1914) 139-146. They do not have any language that this letter demonstrably borrows.

[2] Cf. Dioscorides, *Preface* 6: "Sites are important, whether they are in the mountains, high up, windswept, cold and arid, for the properties of such plants are stronger. Those of plants from flat and wet localities, in the shade and not open to the wind, are generally weaker...." ὡς καὶ παρὰ τὸ ὀρεινοὺς καὶ ὑψηλοὺς καὶ διαπνεομένους καὶ ψυχροὺς καὶ ἀνύδρους εἶναι τοὺς τόπους· ἰσχυρότεραι γάρ εἰσιν αἱ δυνάμεις αὐτῶν. αἱ δὲ ἐν πεδινοῖς καὶ καθύγροις ⟨τόποις⟩ καὶ κατασκίοις καὶ μὴ διαπνεομένοις ἀτονώτεροι κατὰ τὸ πλεῖστον.... The sentiments are the same, but the language differs. (Text from Max Wellmann, *Pedanii Dioscoridis Anazarbei De materia medica* (Berlin: 1907-14), translation from John Scarborough and Vivian Nutton, "The Preface of Dioscorides' Materia Medica: Introduction, Translation, Commentary," *Transactions and Studies of the College of Physicians of Philadelphia* 4 (1982) 187-227.)

ἀλλ' εὐθὺς ἡμῖν ταῦτα πέμψον· καὶ γὰρ ἡ ὥρη τοῦ ἔτεος ἁρμόδιος καὶ ἡ ἀνάγκη τῆς λεγομένης μανίης ἐπείγει. τέχνης δὲ πάσης μὲν ἀλλότριον |
346 ἀναβολή, ἰητρικῆς δὲ καὶ πάνυ, ἐν ᾗ ψυχῆς κίνδυνος ἡ ὑπέρθεσις· ψυχαὶ δὲ τῶν θεραπειῶν οἱ καιροί, ὧν ἡ παραφυλακὴ τὸ τέλος. ἔλπομαι μὲν οὖν ὑγιέα εἶναι τὸν Δημόκριτον καὶ δίχα ἰήσιος. εἰ δ' ἄρα τι σφάλμα φύσιος ἢ καιροῦ ἢ ἄλλης τινὸς αἰτίης γένοιτο, πολλὰ γὰρ ἂν ἡμέας θνητοὺς ἐόντας λάθοι ἅτε μὴ πάγχυ δι' ἀτρεκείης εὐτονέοντας, ἐπὶ τὸ ἄδηλον πᾶσαν χρεὼ δύναμιν ἠθροῖσθαι. οὐ γὰρ ἀρκεῖται ὁ κινδυνεύων οἷσι δυνάμεθα, ἀλλ' ἐπιθυμεῖ καὶ ἃ μὴ δυνάμεθα. καὶ σχεδὸν πρὸς δύο στρατευόμεθα, τὸ μὲν ἀνθρώπου, τὸ δὲ τέχνης, ὧν τὸ μὲν ἄδηλον, τὸ δὲ τῆς ἐπιστήμης ὥρισται. δεῖ δὲ ἐν ἀμφοτέροισι τούτοισι καὶ τύχης. τὸ γὰρ ἀτέκμαρτον ἐν τῇσιν καθάρσεσι δι' εὐλαβείης ἰόντων. καὶ γὰρ στομάχου κάκωσιν ὑφορώμεθα καὶ ξυμμετρίην φαρμακίης πρὸς ἀγνοουμένην φύσιν στοχαζόμεθα. οὐ γὰρ ἡ αὐτὴ καὶ μία φύσις ἁπάντων, ἕτερον δ' αἰεὶ καὶ πρὸς ἑωυτὴν ὁρίζουσα οἰκεῖον. ἐνίοτε δὲ καὶ τῇσι βοτάνῃσιν πολλὰ τῶν ἑρπετῶν ἐνιοβόλησε καὶ περιχανόντα τῇ ἐντὸς αὔρῃ κάκωσιν ἀντ' ἀλεξήσιος αὐτοῖσι προσέπνευσεν. εἰ μή τις ἄρα κηλὶς ἢ σπίλος ἢ ὀδμὴ θηριώδης καὶ ἀπηνὴς τοῦ γενομένου ξύμβολον φανείη, εἶθ' ἡ τέχνη διὰ τὸ ξύμπτωμα τῆς τύχης τῆς κατορθώσιος ἀφήμαρτε. βεβαιότεραι δὲ αἰεὶ αἱ δι' ἐλλεβόρων διὰ τοῦτο καθάρσιές εἰσιν. καὶ Μελάμπους ἐπὶ τῶν Προίτου θυγατέρων καὶ Ἀντικυρεὺς ἐφ' Ἡρακλέους ἱστορέονται |
348 κεχρῆσθαι, μὴ χρησαίμεθα δὲ ἡμεῖς ἐπὶ Δημοκρίτου μηδενὶ τούτων, ἀλλὰ γένοιτο ἐκείνῳ τῶν δραστικωτάτων καὶ ἰητρικωτάτων φαρμάκων σοφίη τέλος. ἔρρωσο.

17. Ἱπποκράτης Δαμαγήτῳ χαίρειν·

Τοῦτ' ἐκεῖνο, Δαμάγητε, ὅπερ εἰκάζομεν, οὐ παρέκοπτεν Δημόκριτος, ἀλλὰ πάντα ὑπερεφρόνει καὶ ἡμέας ἐσωφρόνιζε καὶ δι' ἡμέων πάντας ἀνθρώπους. ἐξέπεμψα δέ σοι, φιλότης, ὡς ἀληθέως τὴν Ἀσκληπιάδα νῆα, ἣν πρόες μετὰ τοῦ Ἁλίου ἐπίσημον καὶ Ὑγιείην, ἐπεὶ κατὰ δαίμονα τῷ ἔοντι ἱστιοδρόμηκε καὶ ἐκείνῃ τῇ ἡμέρῃ κατέπλευσεν ἐς Ἄβδηρα, ᾗπερ αὐτοῖσιν ἐπεστάλκειν ἀφίξεσθαι. πάντας οὖν ἀλέας πρὸ τῶν πυλέων εὕρομεν ὡς εἰκὸς ἡμέας περιμένοντας, οὐκ ἄνδρας μούνους, ἀλλὰ καὶ γυναῖκας, ἔτι δὲ καὶ πρεσβύτας καὶ παιδία, νὴ θεούς, κατηφέας, καὶ τὰ

---

2 τέχνης μὲν γὰρ πάσης U ‖ 3 ψυχαί: ψυχῆς U ‖ 5 ὑγιέα εἶναι: ὑγιαίνειν U τὸν om. O ἄρα om. U ‖ 6 ἄλλως U ἄλλη τις αἰτίη O ἂν om. MVb ‖ 7 δι' ἀτρεκείης: μηδ' ἀτρεκίης O ‖ 8 χρέο MV ‖ 9 post σχέδον add. ἀεὶ UbO post στρατ. add. τέλεα UbO ‖ 12 δι' εὐλαβίης τοῖσιν ἢ ᾗ πόοις καὶ γὰρ καὶ στομάχου U κάκωσιν: κάθαρσιν O ‖ 14 φύσις: στάσις U ἴασις b (corr. b^2) αἰεί: εἰ M καὶ^{II} om. bO ‖ 15 οἰκειοῖ M post δὲ add. τὸ πᾶν ἀπώλεσεν b ‖ 17 ἀλέξιος O post προσεπν. add. καὶ τούτου ἄγνοια ἔσται U ‖ 20 διὰ τοῦτο om. U εἰσιν om. O ante καὶ add. αἷς bO ‖ 22 μὴ om. U ‖ 23 ἐκείνων b τὰ δραστικώτατα τῶν φαρμάκων U καὶ ἰητρ. om. UO σοφίης U$M^2$$b^2$ ‖ 24 τέλος. ἔρρωσο om. O ‖ 26 τουτ': τοῦτο ἦν U ‖ 27 πάντα: πάντας O πάντα corr. in πάντας b post ἡμέων iterum ἐσωφρόνιζε add. O ‖ 28 ἐξεπέμψαμεν b^2U ‖ 29 ἥν: ἣ U ᾗ bO πρόες: πρόσθε M πρόθες b πρόσθες O πρότερον U ὑγιῆ MUV ‖ 31 ἀολλέας UbO ‖ 32 μοῦνον UO ‖ 33 καὶ post δὲ om. Vb ἠηθέους VM (corr. M^2) νὴ τοὺς θεοὺς O κατηφέα MUbO καὶ om. MO

flowers (you call them spring-flowers), which I consider weak, slack, and of sweet juice. All that have flowing juice or sap should be brought in glass jars, and bring the leaves, blossoms and roots in new cups that are bound tightly so that they will not be open to the winds and lose their concentration of pharmaceutical virtue so as to faint, as it were, dead away.[1] But, send these things to us immediately. The time of year is fitting and the constraints of the so-called madness press. Delay is foreign to all science, especially to medicine in which postponement is danger to life. The soul of therapy is in opportunity, and our job is to be on guard for opportunities.[2] *Aphorisms*:1.1 I hope that Democritus is well, even without treatment. But if there should be some failure of nature or of opportunity or of some other cause (many things could escape our notice, since we are mortals whose exertions are not always precise), we must gather all our force against what is obscure. The man in danger is not satisfied with what we can do. He wants also what we cannot. It is almost as though we go to combat with two things, the human being and science, the first obscure and the second limited by what we know. In both of them we have need of luck. Take, as an example, the lack of precise standards in purgation for those who proceed with caution: we anticipate harm to the stomach, and we aim at equating the pharmaceutical effect with the unknown nature. One and the same constitution does not belong to everyone, and it is always defining something different as appropriate for itself. Sometimes, too, in the case of plants, many snakes have injected their poison into them, and gaping around them, have, with their inner fumes, breathed harmfulness into them instead of helpfulness.[3] Hence, if no stain or blemish or foul animal odor appears as token of what has happened, the science, because of the hazards of fortune, then fails of correct procedure. Therefore, catharsis with the hellebores is more certain. Melampus is famous for having used it for the daughters of Proetus, and Anticyreus for Heracles, but I hope we use none of these things on Democritus! May wisdom in the end be among the most effective and healing drugs for him. Be well!

17. Hippocrates to Damagetus. Greetings.

Just as we conjectured, Damagetus, Democritus was not demented, but was very wise in all things, and he gave me instruction in virtue, and through me all men. I have sent you back the ship, my dear friend. /How truly it was Asclepius'

---

[1] These are standard procedures and common containers for storing medical material. Dioscorides, *Preface* 9, recommends limewood boxes, papyrus, and silver, glass, horn, earthenware, boxwood, copper, and tin containers for the various types of drugs.

[2] This may allude to *Precepts* 1, "Opportunity is that in which there is little time" (καιρὸς ἐν ᾧ χρόνος οὐ πολύς) or *Precepts* may allude to this passage if it was written later. Both are probably aware of *Aphorisms* 1. 1, "Opportunity is fleeting" (καιρὸς ὀξύς).

[3] The baleful effect of snakes on plants is accepted by the pharmacologists. Poisonous mushrooms are so because they have absorbed snake breath or venom at the snake's lair: Dioscorides *Materia Medica* 4.82, Nicander, *Alexipharmaka* 521-6. Pliny, N.H. 22.95, extends the notion to many plants.

νήπια· καὶ οὗτοι μέντοι ὡς ἐπὶ μαινομένῳ τῷ Δημοκρίτῳ, ὁ δὲ μετ'
ἀκριβείης τότε ὑπερεφιλοσόφει. ἐπεὶ δέ με εἶδον, ἔδοξάν που σμικρὸν ἐφ'
350 ἑωυτῶν γεγονέναι καὶ χρηστὰς ἐλπίδας ἐποιοῦντο. ὁ δὲ Φιλοποίμην
ἄγειν ἐπὶ τὴν ξεινίην με ὥρμητο κἀκείνοισι ξυνεδόκει τοῦτο. ἐγὼ δέ, Ὦ
ἄνδρες, ἔφην, Ἀβδηρῖται, οὐδέν ἐστί μοι προὔργου ἢ Δημόκριτον θεήσασθαι.
οἱ δ' ἐπῄνουν ἀκούσαντες καὶ ἥσθησαν, ἦγόν τε με | ξυντόμως διὰ τῆς
ἀγορῆς, οἱ μὲν ἑπόμενοι, οἱ δὲ προθέοντες ἑτέρωθεν ἕτεροι, Σῷζε, λέγοντες,
βοήθει, θεράπευσον. κἀγὼ παρῄνεον θαρρεῖν ὡς τάχα μὲν οὐδενὸς ἐόντος
κακοῦ, πίσυνος ἐτησίῃσιν ὥρῃσιν, εἰ δ' ἄρα καί τινος, βραχέος,
εὐδιορθώτου.

2. Καὶ ἅμα ταῦτα λέγων ᾔειν. οὐδὲ γὰρ πόρρω ἦν ἡ οἰκίη, μᾶλλον δ'
οὐδ' ἡ πόλις ὅλη. παρῆμεν οὖν, πλησίον γὰρ τοῦ τείχους ἐτύγχανε, καὶ
ἀνάγουσίν με ἡσυχῇ· ἔπειτα κατόπιν τοῦ πύργου βουνὸς ἦν τις ὑψηλός,
μακρῇσι καὶ λασίῃσιν αἰγείροισιν ἐπίσκιος, ἔνθεν τε ἐθεωρεῖτο τὰ τοῦ
Δημοκρίτου καταγώγια. καὶ αὐτὸς ὁ Δημόκριτος καθῆστο ὑπό τινι
ἀμφιλαφεῖ καὶ χθαμαλῇ πλατανίστῳ, ἐν ἐξωμίδι παχείῃ, μοῦνος,
ἀνείληφος, ἐπὶ λιθίνῳ θώκῳ, ὠχριακὼς πάνυ καὶ λιπόσαρκος, κουριῶν τὰ
γένεια. παρ' αὐτὸν δ' ἐπὶ δεξιῆς λεπτόρρυτον ὕδωρ κατὰ πρηνοῦς τοῦ
λόφου ἠρεμαίως ἐκελάρυζεν. ἦν δέ τι τέμενος ὑπὲρ ἐκεῖνον τὸν λόφον, ὡς
ἐν ὑπονοίῃ κατεικάζοντι, νυμφέων ἱδρυμένον, αὐτοφυτοῖσιν ἐπηρεφὲς
352 ἀμπέλοισιν. ὁ δ' εἶχεν ἐν εὐκοσμίῃ πολλῇ ἐπὶ τοῖν γονάτοιν βιβλίον, καὶ
ἕτερα δέ τινα ἐξ ἀμφοῖν τοῖν μεροῖν αὐτῷ παρεβέβλητο· σεσώρευντο δὲ
καὶ ζῷα συχνὰ ἀνατετμημένα δι' ὅλων. ὁ δὲ ὁτὲ μὲν ξυντόνως ἔγραφεν
ἐγκείμενος, ὁτὲ δὲ ἠρέμει πάμπολύ | τι ἐπέχων καὶ ἐν ἑωυτῷ μερμηρίζων.
εἶτα μετ' οὐ πολὺ τούτων ἐρδομένων ἐξαναστὰς περιεπάτει καὶ τὰ
σπλάγχνα τῶν ζῴων ἐπεσκόπει καὶ καταθεὶς αὐτὰ μετελθὼν
ἐκαθέζετο. οἱ δὲ Ἀβδηρῖται περιεστῶτές με κατηφεῖς καὶ οὐ πόρρω τὰς
ὄψεις δακρυόντων ἔχοντές φασιν, Ὁρῇς μέντοι τὸν Δημοκρίτου βίον, ὦ
Ἱππόκρατες, ὡς μέμηνεν καὶ οὔτε ὅτι θέλει οἶδεν οὔτε ὅτι ἔρδει; καί τις
αὐτῶν ἔτι μᾶλλον ἐνδείξασθαι βουλόμενος τὴν μανίην αὐτοῦ, ὀξὺ
ἀνεκώκυσεν εἴκελον γυναικὶ ἐπὶ θανάτῳ τέκνου ὀδυρομένῃ· εἶτ'
ἀνῴμωξεν ὑποκρινόμενος παροδίτην ἄλλος ὀλέσαντα ὃ διεκόμιζεν. καὶ ὁ

---

1 ante ὡς add. ὧδε εἶχον OM² post Δημοκ. add. ὧδε εἶχον U || 2 που om. O post που add. ἡδίους b || 2-3 μικρόν τι ἐφ ἑωυτοῖσι b || 4 με post ἄγειν O || 4-5 ἐγὼ δὲ ἔφην ὦ ἀβδηρ. (om. ἄνδρες) O || 6 ἦγοντο δὲ V ἦγόν τε MO ἦγόν τε αὐτῶν b || 7 Σῷζε: ὦ Ζεῦ M² ὦ Ζεῦ βασιλεῦ cd βασιλεῦ a || 8 παρηγόρουν bO ἐόντος om. O || 10 ante εὐδιορθ. add καὶ. U || 11 ἡ οἰκίη: ἡ κίη U || 12 ὅλη om. O γὰρ: δὲ Vb || 13 ἡσυχίῃ O τις ἦν O || 14 δασῇσιν MV ἐντεῦθεν Ub (corr. b²) ἐθεωρεῖτο: ἑωρᾶτο O || 15 ἐκάθητο UO || 17 ἀνήλιπος Ub (corr. b²) ἀνήληφος M² et in marg., ἐκτετηγμένος ἢ ἀνυπόδητος || 19 post λόφου add. θέον b ὑπερκείμενον U || 20 ἐπιρρεφὲς MVb || 21 τῶν γονάτων U || 22 αὐτοῦ U παρεμβεβέβλητο U σεσώρευτο bO ἐσεστώρευντο U || 23 συντόμως O || 24 τι: τε O ante ἐν add ἦν. b || 25 ante ἐρδ. add. τῶν b || 26 περιεσκόπεε O || 27 ante ἐκαθέζ. add. πάλιν. U με om. M (corr. M²) || 28 δακρύων O ante Δημοκ. add. τοῦ O ante ὦ add. αὐτὸς b || 28-9 ὦ Ἱππ. post μέμηνεν O ὅτι ἔρδει: ὃ ἔρδει O || 30 ἔτι om. O τὴν μανίην ante βουλ. U αὐτοῦ om. b (corr. b²) || 31 ἐκώκυσεν O ὀλοφυρομένῃ UbO || 32 ante ὑποκριν. add. πάλιν U πάλιν ἄλλος b ἄλλος: ἄλλον U om. b ἀπωλεσάντα b ὃ: τι ὧν U ὃν O τι ὧν δ' ἂν b om. M

ship! Put the device of Hygieia on her next to that of Helios,[1] since she truly sailed with a god/and put in to Abdera on the very day I had told them I would arrive.

We found them all gathered before the gates, apparently waiting for us, not men only but women, too, and old men and children, dreadfully disheartened, even the infants; they came for the sake of a maddened Democritus, while he was even at that moment doing precise higher philosophy. When they saw me they seemed to become somewhat composed, and they affected optimism. Philopoimen started to lead me off to my guest quarters and they approved. But I said, "Men of Abdera, for me nothing is more important than to see Democritus." When they heard it they praised me and were cheered up. And they led me immediately off through the agora, some behind, some preceding on both sides, saying "Save him, help him, heal him." I advised them to be of good cheer, since perhaps there was nothing wrong, and trusting the season of the Etesian winds, if there was something it was perhaps brief, easily mended.

2. Talking thus I went along, for his house was not far; indeed, the whole city was not. Then we were there, for it was near the wall and they brought me forward quietly. After that, behind the tower, there was a high hill shaded by great shaggy poplars, and from that spot one looked down on the residence of Democritus. And Democritus himself was sitting under a spreading low plane tree, in a coarse shirt, alone, not anointed with oil, on a stone seat, pale and emaciated, with untrimmed beard. Next to him on the right a small stream bubbled down the hill's slope softly. There was a sanctuary on top of that hill, which I conjectured was dedicated to the nymphs, roofed over with wild grapes. He had a papyrus roll on his knees in a very neat manner, and some other book-rolls were laid out on both sides. And stacked around were a large number of animals, generally cut up. He sometimes bent and applied himself intensely to writing, sometimes he sat quietly attentive, pondering within himself. Then after a short time of this activity he stood up and walked around and examined the entrails of the animals, set them down and went back and sat down. The Abderites, standing about me downcast, their eyes not far from tears, said, "You see Democritus' way of life, Hippocrates, how mad he is, how he doesn't know what he wants or what he is doing? One man, who wanted even more to point out his madness wailed shrilly like a woman lamenting a child's death. Then another groaned imitating a wayfarer who had lost his belongings. When

[1] Lionel Casson, *Ships and Seamanship in the Ancient World* , 346 n. 7, suggests that Helios is thought of as the equivalent of Apollo, father of Asclepius, and proposes that the ship's "device" (*episemon*) somewhere included Asclepius in the decoration. That may be what the author is imagining, although Helios is nowhere called Asclepius' father that I have seen.

Δημόκριτος ὑπακούων τὰ μὲν ἐμειδία, τὰ δὲ ἐξεγέλα καὶ οὐκέτι οὐδὲν ἔγραφε, τὴν δὲ κεφαλὴν θαμινὰ ἐπέσειεν. ἐγὼ δέ, Ὑμεῖς μέν, ἔφην, Ἀβδηρῖται, αὐτόθι μίμνετε· ἐγγυτέρω δ' αὐτὸς καὶ λόγων καὶ σωμάτων τἀνδρὸς γενηθεὶς ἰδών τε καὶ ἀκούσας εἴσομαι τοῦ πάθους τὴν ἀλήθειαν.

3. Καὶ ταῦτ' εἰπὼν κατέβαινον ἡσυχῇ. ἦν δὲ ὀξὺ καὶ ἐπίφορον ἐκεῖνο τὸ χωρίον· μόγις οὖν διαστηριζόμενος διῆλθον. ἐπεὶ δ' ἐπλησίαζον, ἔτυχεν ἐπελθὸν αὐτῷ ὅτι δήποτε γράφειν ἐνθουσιωδῶς καὶ μεθ' ὁρμῆς· εἰστήκειν οὖν περιμένων αὐτοῦ τὸν καιρὸν τῆς ἀναπαύσιος· ὁ δὲ μετὰ σμικρὸν τῆς φορῆς λήξας τοῦ γραφείου ἀνέβλεψέν τε ἐς ἐμὲ προσιόντα καί φησιν,
354 Χαῖρε, ξεῖνε. κἀγώ, Πολλά γε καὶ σύ, Δημόκριτε, ἀνδρῶν σοφώτατε. | ὁ δὲ αἰδεσθείς, οἶμαι, ὅτι ὀνομαστὶ μὴ προσεῖπέν με, Σὲ δέ, ἔφη, τί καλέομεν; ἄγνοια γὰρ τοῦ σοῦ ὀνόματος ἦν ἡ τοῦ ξείνου προσηγορίη. Ἱπποκράτης, ἔφην, ἔμοιγε τοὔνομα, ὁ ἰητρός. ὁ δὲ εἶπεν, Ἡ τῶν Ἀσκληπιαδῶν εὐγένεια· πολύ γε σοῦ τὸ κλέος τῆς ἐν ἰητρικῇ σοφίης πεφοίτηκεν καὶ ἐς ἡμέας ἀφῖκται· τί δὲ χρέος, ἑταῖρε, δεῦρό σε ἤγαγε; μᾶλλον δὲ πρὸ πάντων κάθησο. ὁρῇς δὲ ὡς ἔστιν οὗτος οὐκ ἀηδὴς φύλλων θῶκος, χλοερὸς καὶ μαλακὸς ἐγκαθίσαι, προσηνέστερος τῶν τῆς τύχης ἐπιφθόνων θώκων. καθίσαντος δέ μου πάλιν φησίν. Ἴδιον οὖν ἢ ἐπιδήμιον πρῆγμα διζήμενος δεῦρο ἀφῖξαι; φράζε σαφῶς. καὶ γὰρ ἡμεῖς ὅτι δυναίμεθα συνεργοῖμεν ἄν. κἀγώ, Τὸ μὲν κατ' ἀληθείην, ἔφην, αἴτιον, σέο δεῦρο χάριν ἥκω ξυντυχεῖν σοφῷ ἀνδρί· ἔχει δὲ πρόφασιν ἡ πατρίς, ἧς πρεσβείην τελέω. ὁ δέ, Ξεινίῃ τοίνυν, φησί, τὰ πρῶτα κέχρησο ἡμετέρῃ. πειρώμενος δὲ κἀγὼ κατὰ πάντα τἀνδρὸς καίπερ ἤδη μοι δήλου μὴ παρακόπτειν ἐνέοντος, Φιλοποίμενα οἶσθα, ἔφην, πολίτην ἐόντα ὑμέτερον; ὁ δέ, Καὶ μάλα, εἶπεν, τὸν Δάμωνος λέγεις υἱὸν τὸν οἰκοῦντα παρὰ τὴν Ἑρμαΐδα κρήνην; Τοῦτον, εἶπον, ᾧ καὶ τυγχάνω ἐκ πατέρων ἴδιος ξεῖνος· ἀλλὰ σύ, Δημόκριτε, τῇ
356 κρείσσονί με ξεινίῃ δέχου. καὶ πρῶτόν γε τί ἦν τοῦτο ὃ γράφεις, φράζε. | ὁ δ' ἐπισχὼν ὀλίγον, Περὶ μανίης, ἔφη. κἀγώ, Ὦ Ζεῦ βασιλεῦ, φημί, εὐκαίρως γε ἀντιγράφεις πρὸς τὴν πόλιν. ὁ δέ, Ποίην, φησίν, πόλιν,

---

1 ἐπακούων UO καὶ om. O ‖ 2 γράφων O ‖ 3 ante Ἀβδ. add. ὦ O μείνατε UO καὶ σώματος καὶ λόγων b καὶ λόγου καὶ σώματος O ‖ 3-4 καὶ λόγων τἀνδρὸς καὶ σωμάτων γενήσομαι καὶ ἀκριβέστερον ἰδὸν καὶ U τε om. O ‖ 6 ante οὖν add. δ' O ‖ 7 ἐπελθὼν MUVa τότε ἐπελθὸν cd ὅτε ἐπῆλθον b (corr. b^2) ‖ 8 αὐτοῦ post καιρὸν U ‖ 8-9 τῆς φορῆς post γραφείου U, post λήξας bV ‖ 9 γράφειν Ob (corr. b^2) ἐνέβλεψε Vb προσέβλεψε O προσιόντα post φησιν V ‖ 10 γε: δὲ O Δημ. post σοφωτ. U ‖ 11 ὀνόματι U ὀνομά τι b (corr. b^2) μοι V τί: τίνα O καλέωμεν V ‖ 12 ἀγνοίαι b ἦν om. O habent πρόφασις post ὀνόματος MUVO post ἦν b seclusi οὔνομα O ‖ 13 ὁ δὲ om. b ‖ 14 ἐν ἰητρικῇ: ἰητρικῆς Ua ‖ 14-15 καὶ...ἀφῖκται: ὡς ἐμὲ O ‖ 15 σε ante χρέος UbO ἑταῖρε post ἤγαγε O ‖ 16 κάθισον O κάθησιν U ὡς... θῶκος: τὸν οὕτως ουκ ἀηδῆ φύλλων θημῶνα ὡς O θῶκος ante φύλλων V ante χλοερὸς add. ὅτι M, ἔτι U ‖ 17 ἐγκαθίσαι: ἐστι καθίσαι O τῆς om. bO ψυχῆς M ‖ 18 πάλιν: αὖτις b ἴδιόν τι ἢ δήμιον U τι post οὖν add. bO πρῆγμα post διζήμενος UbO ‖ 19 ἄν .om. UO ‖ 20 αἴτιον om. O σέο et χάριν om. U σεο κτλ: ἕνεκα σεῦ· δεῦρο γὰρ ἥκω σοι συντυχεῖν ἀνδρὶ σοφῷ O ‖ 21 σὴν πρεσβείαν τελέως U | 22 φησί om. O κἀγὼ: ἐγὼ b om. O ‖ 23 καταδήλου U ἐνέοντος: ἐόντος Ub om. O ‖ 24 πολιήτην ὑμετ. ἐόντα b εἶπεν: ἔφη εἰ O ‖ 26 ᾧ: οὗ MU ἴδιος: φίλιος b ἰδιόξενος Ob^2 ‖ 27 γ' ἔτι ἦν M ἦν om. U . ὃ om M γράφεις: γράφων τυγχάνεις MUbO ‖ 28 post ὀλίγον add. χρόνον b Ὦ om. O ‖ 29 γράφεις U πρὸς om. b (corr. b^2) φησίν: φὴ U

Democritus heard the first he smiled, on hearing the second, he laughed. He stopped writing, and shook his head frequently. I said, "Abderites, you stay here. When I have got nearer to his speech and his person and have seen and heard him I shall know the truth of his affection."

3. So saying I descended quietly. The place sloped sharply to a point, so that I hardly kept my footing as I proceeded. And when I was coming near, it happened that there had come on him a fit of writing something with inspired intensity. I stood and waited for the opportunity of his pausing. And he, after a short time, stopped the movement of his pen, glanced up as I approached, and said, "Greetings, stranger." And I, "Many greetings to you, Democritus, wisest of men." He, embarrassed, I think, that he had not addressed me by name, "And you, how shall we address you? My calling you 'stranger' was ignorance of your name." "Hippocrates is my name," I said, "the physician." And he said, "The excellence of the Asclepiads! The great fame of your wisdom in medicine has traveled far, and has reached even us. But what brings you here, my friend? But do first take a seat. You see how pleasant is this seat of leaves here, green and soft for sitting, more soothing than thrones of those envied for their fortune." I sat and he spoke again: "Do you come in pursuit of private business or public? Tell me plainly, for if I could be of any help, I would." And I said, "The real reason is that I came here because of you, to meet a wise man. But the excuse was offered by the fatherland whose embassage I perform." And he, "First of all, take advantage of my entertainment." And making test of the man in all ways, though it was already obvious to me that he was not really mad, I said, "Do you know Philopoimen, your fellow townsman?" And he, "Indeed. You mean Damon's son who lives by the fountain of Hermes?" "That is he," I said. "I am his proper guest by ancestral connection. But you, Democritus, please accept me in still greater guest-frendship, and first tell me what it is that you are writing?" After hesitating briefly, he said, "A treatise on madness." And I, "Oh Zeus, King of the gods! You are writing a timely refutation of the city!" And he, "City?

Ἱππόκρατες; ἐγὼ δέ, Οὐδέν, ἔφην, ὦ Δημόκριτε, ἀλλ' οὐκ οἶδ' ὅκως προὔπεσεν. ἀλλὰ τί περὶ μανίης γράφεις; Τί γάρ, εἶπεν, ἄλλο ἢ τίς πέλει καὶ ὅκως ἀνθρώποισιν ἐγγίνεται καὶ τίνα τρόπον ἀπολωφέοιτο. τά τε γὰρ ζῷα, ἔφη, ταῦτα ὁκόσα ὁρῇς, τούτου μέντοι γε οὕνεκα ἀνατέμνω, οὐ μισέων θεοῦ ἔργα, χολῆς δὲ διζήμενος φύσιν καὶ θέσιν. οἶσθα γὰρ ἀνθρώπων παρακοπῆς ὡς αἰτίη ἐπὶ τὸ πολὺ αὕτη πλεονάσασα, ἐπεὶ πᾶσι μὲν φύσει ἐνυπάρχει, ἀλλὰ παρ' οἷσι μὲν ἐλάσσων, παρ' οἷσι δέ τι πλείων. ἡ δ' ἀμετρίη αὐτῆς νοῦσοι τυγχάνουσιν, ὡς ὕλης ὁτὲ μὲν ἀγαθῆς, ὁτὲ δὲ φαύλης ὑποκειμένης. κἀγώ, Νὴ Δία, ἔφην, ὦ Δημόκριτε, ἀληθέως γε καὶ φρονίμως λέγεις· ὅθεν εὐδαίμονά σε κρίνω τοσαύτης ἀπολαύοντα ἡσυχίης. ἡμῖν δὲ μετέχειν ταύτης οὐκ ἐπιτέτραπται. ἐρεομένου δέ, Διὰ τί, ὦ Ἱππόκρατες, οὐκ ἐπιτέτραπται; Ὅτι, ἔφην, ἢ ἀποικίη ἢ τέκνα ἢ δάνεια ἢ νοῦσοι ἢ θάνατοι ἢ δμῶες ἢ γάμοι ἢ τοιαῦτά τινα τὴν εὐκαιρίην ὑποτάμνεται.

4. Ἐνταῦθα δὴ ὁ ἀνὴρ ἐς τὸ εἰωθὸς κατηνέχθη καὶ μάλα ἀθροῦν τι ἀνεκάγχασε καὶ ἐπετώθασε καὶ τὸ λοιπὸν ἡσυχίην ἦγε. κἀγώ, Τί μέντοι,
358 Δημόκριτε, ἔφην, γελᾷς; | πότερον τὰ ἀγαθὰ ὧν εἶπον ἢ τὰ κακά; ὁ δὲ ἔτι μᾶλλον ἐγέλα. καὶ ἄπωθεν ὁρεῦντες οἱ Ἀβδηρῖται οἱ μὲν τὰς κεφαλὰς αὐτῶν ἔπαιον, οἱ δὲ τὰ μέτωπα, οἱ δὲ τὰς τρίχας ἔτιλλον. καὶ γάρ, ὡς ὕστερον ἔφησαν, πλεονάζοντι παρὰ τὸ εἰωθὸς ἐχρήσατο τῷ γέλωτι. ὑποτυχὼν δ' ἐγώ, Ἀλλὰ μήν, ἔφην, σοφῶν ἄριστε, Δημόκριτε, ποθέω γὰρ αἰτίην τοῦ περὶ σὲ πάθεος καταλαβέσθαι, τίνος ἄξιος ἐφάνην ἐγὼ γέλωτος ἢ τὰ λεχθέντα ὅκως μαθὼν παύσωμαι τῆς αἰτίης ἢ σὺ ἐλεγχθεὶς διακρούσῃ τοὺς ἀκαίρους γέλωτας. ὁ δέ, Ἡράκλεις, ἔφη, εἰ γὰρ δυνήσῃ με ἐλέγξαι, θεραπείην θεραπεύσεις οἵην οὐδένα πώποτε, Ἱππόκρατες. Καὶ πῶς οὐκ ἐλεγχθείσῃ, ἔφην, ὦ ἄριστε; ἢ οὐκ οἴει ἄτοπός γε εἶναι γελῶν ἀνθρώπου θάνατον ἢ νοῦσον ἢ παρακοπὴν ἢ μανίην ἢ μελαγχολίην ἢ σφαγὴν ἢ ἄλλο τι χέρειον ἢ τοὔμπαλιν γάμους ἢ πανηγύριας ἢ τεκνογονίην ἢ μυστήρια ἢ ἀρχὰς καὶ τιμὰς ἢ ἄλλο τι ὅλως ἀγαθόν; καὶ γὰρ ἃ δέον οἰκτείρειν γελῇς καὶ ἐφ' οἷσιν ἥδεσθαι χρή, καταγελᾷς τούτων, ὥστε μήτε ἀγαθὸν μήτε κακὸν παρά σοι

---

1 post ὅκως add. ἔφην b ‖ 2 προὔπεσον Ob^2 πρὸς ἔπεσεν U ἢ τίς πέλει: O πλὴν εἴ τις εἴη VMb πλὴν ἥτις εἴη U ‖ 3 ἀπόλοιτο M τε om. UO ‖ 4 ταῦτα ἔφη U ‖ 6 ἐπὶ πολὺ bO ἐπὶ πάσῃ U ‖ 7 ἔλαττον M ‖ 8 αἱ δ' ἀμετρίαι U ‖ 8-9 ποτὲ...ποτὲ U ‖ 9 φλαύρης b ‖ 10 γε: τε O βάζεις corr. in λέγεις b ἀπολαύοντα τοσαύτης O ‖ 11 ἐπιτρέπεται b ἐρωμένου U ἐρομένου VbO διότι V ‖ 11-12 ἐρεομένου...οὐκ om. a ‖ 12 ὦ om. O ἢ^1: ἡ V ἀποικίη: ἄγροι ἢ οἰκίη b ἀγροικίη M ‖ 14 ἡμῶν ἀποτέμνεται U ὑποτάμνει b (corr. b^2) ‖ 15 post εἰωθὸς add. πάθος UbO ‖ 16 καὶ ἀνακαγχάσαι καὶ ἐπετωθάσαι M ‖ 17 Δημόκριτε, ἔφην: ὦ Δημ. ἔφην b ἔφην ὦ Δημ. UO φλαῦρα b (corr. b^2) ‖ 18 καὶ om. b ‖ 18-19 οἱ μὲν...ἔτιλλον post γέλωτι (20) V ‖ 19 post τρίχας add. αὐτῶν O ‖ 20 ἆθος corr. in εἰωθὸς b post εἰωθὸς add. κατηνέχθη καὶ μάλ' ἄθρουν τι O ‖ 21 ἔφην ante ἀλλὰ O ‖ 22-3 ἐφάνην post γέλωτος V ἄξιος post γέλωτος b ‖ 23 post γέλωτος add. αὐτὸς O λαληθέντα O post ὅκως add. ἢ bO παύσομαι MbO σὺ om. M ‖ 24 εὐκαίρους U ‖ 25 οὐδεπώποτε MU ‖ 26 ante Ἱππ. add. ὦ O ἐλεγχθείης MO οἶσθα O ‖ 27 θάνατον ἀνθρ. O παρακοὴν U ‖ 27-8 ἢ μανίην ἢ μελαγχολίην om. O ‖ 28 χεῖρον MU ‖ 29 καί: ἢ bO ‖ 29-30 ἄλλο τι ὅλως: πᾶν ὅλως ὄνομα O ἄλλο τι πᾶν ὅλως b ‖ 31 μήτε ἀγαθὸν om. U

What do you mean, Hippocrates?" And I, "Nothing, Democritus. That slipped out somehow. But what are you writing on madness?" "Just what it is, how it comes on men, and how to relieve it. All these animals that you see here I am dissecting for that, not because I hate divine works, but because I am pursuing the nature and location of the gall. You know how its overabundance generally causes dementia in men, since it is present by nature in all but less in some and somewhat more in others. Disproportion of it becomes disease because it is a substance sometimes good, sometimes harmful." And I said, "By Zeus, Democritus, you speak truly and wisely. For that reason I consider you blessed to enjoy such leisure. It has not fallen to me to share in it." And when he asked, "Why, Hippocrates, has it not so fallen?" "Because," I said, "traveling, children, debts, disease, death, servants, marriages: such things whittle away my leisure."

4. Thereupon the man was swept back to his usual manner. He burst out laughing; he scoffed and then remained silent. I said, "But what are you laughing at, Democritus, the good things I mentioned, or the bad ones?" He laughed even more, and looking on from a distance some of the Abderites struck their heads, some their foreheads, some pulled out their hair because as they later said, he was laughing more excessively than usual. I interrupted him and said, "But, Democritus, wisest of men, I want to find out the reason for your affection, why I or what I said seems to deserve laughter, so that, when I find out, I can cure my fault, or you, when you are proved mistaken, can repress your inappropriate laughter." He said, "By Heracles, if you can prove me mistaken you will have effected a cure such as you have never achieved for anyone, Hippocrates." "How shall you not be proved mistaken, oh best of men?" I said. "Don't you think you are outlandish to laugh at a man's death or illness, or delusion, or madness, or melancholy, murder, or something still worse, or again at marriages, feasts, births, initiations, offices and honors, or anything else wholly good? Things that demand grief you laugh at, and when things should bring happiness you laugh at them. There is no distinction between good and bad with you." And he said,

διακεκρίσθαι. ὁ δέ, Ταῦτα μὲν εὖ, ἔφη, λέγεις, ὦ Ἱππόκρατες, ἀλλ' οὐκ οἶσθά πω τοῦ ἡμετέρου γέλωτος αἰτίην· μαθὼν δ' εὖ οἶδ' ὅτι κρέσσονα τῆς πρεσβείης ἀντιφορτισάμενος ἀποίσεις θεραπείην τὸν ἐμὸν γέλωτα τῇ πατρίδι καὶ ἑωυτῷ καὶ τοὺς ἄλλους δυνήσῃ σωφρονίζειν· ἀνθ' ὧν ἴσως κἀμὲ διδάξεις ἰητρικὴν ἀμοιβηδόν, γνοὺς ὅσῃ σπουδῇ περὶ τὰ ἀσπούδαστα
360 φιλοτιμεύμενοι | πρήσσειν τὰ μηδενὸς ἄξια πάντες ἄνθρωποι τὸν βίον ἀναλίσκουσι, γελώτων ἄξια διοικεῦντες. ἐγὼ δέ, Λέγε, φημί, πρὸς θεῶν, μήποτε γὰρ διαλανθάνει πᾶς ὁ κόσμος νοσέων καὶ οὐκ ἔχει ὅκου διαπέμψηται πρεσβείην πρὸς θεραπείην· τί γὰρ ἂν εἴη ἔξω αὐτοῦ; ὁ δ' ὑπολαβών, Πολλαί γε, φησίν, ἀπειρίαι κόσμων εἰσίν, Ἱππόκρατες, καὶ μηδαμῶς, ἑταῖρε, κατασμικρολόγει πλουσίην τὴν φύσιν ἐοῦσαν. Ἀλλὰ ταῦτα μέν, ἔφην, Δημόκριτε, διδάξεις ἐν ἰδίῳ καιρῷ. εὐλαβοῦμαι γὰρ μή πως καὶ τὴν ἀπειρίην διεξιὼν γελῆν ἄρξῃ· ἴσθι δὲ νῦν περὶ τοῦ σοῦ γέλωτος τῷ βίῳ λόγον δώσων.

5. Ὁ δὲ μάλα τρανὸν ἀπιδών μοι, Δύο, φησί, τοῦ ἐμοῦ γέλωτος αἰτίας δοκεῖς, ἀγαθὰ καὶ φαῦλα· ἐγὼ δὲ ἕνα γελῶ τὸν ἄνθρωπον, ἀνοίης μὲν γέμοντα, κενεὸν δὲ πρηγμάτων ὀρθῶν, πάσῃσιν ἐπιβολῇσιν νηπιάζοντα καὶ μηδεμιῆς ἕνεκεν ὠφελείης ἀλγέοντα τοὺς ἀνηνύτους μόχθους, πείρατα γῆς καὶ ἀορίστους μυχοὺς ἀμετρίῃσιν ἐπιθυμίῃσιν ὁδεύοντα, ἄργυρον τήκοντα καὶ χρυσὸν καὶ μὴ παυόμενον τῆς κτήσιος ταύτης, αἰεὶ δὲ θορυβεύμενον περὶ τὸ πλέον, ὅκως αὐτὸς ἐλάσσων γένηται· καὶ οὐδὲ αἰσχύνεται λεγόμενος εὐδαίμων, ὅτι χάσματα γῆς ὀρύσσει δεσμίων χερσίν,
362 ὧν οἱ μὲν ὑπὸ σομφῆς ἐπιπεσούσης τῆς γῆς | ἐφθάρησαν, οἱ δὲ πολυχρονιωτάτην ἔχοντες τὴν ἀνάγκην ὡς ἐν πατρίδι τῇ κολάσει παραμένουσιν, ἄργυρον καὶ χρυσὸν μαστεύοντες, ἴχνη κόνεως καὶ ψήγματα ἐρευνῶντες, ψάμμον ἄλλην ἀλλαχόθεν ἀγείροντες καὶ τῆς γῆς φλέβας ἐκτέμνοντες ἐς περιουσίην, αἰεὶ βωλοποιεῦντες ἐκ γῆς μητρός. τὸ δὲ μίαν γῆν καὶ τὴν αὐτὴν ἐοῦσαν καὶ θαυμάζοντες πατοῦσιν· ὅσος γέλως· ἐπιμόχθου καὶ κρυφίης γῆς ἐρῶσι τὴν φανερὴν ὑβρίζοντες. κύνας ὠνεῦνται, οἱ δ' ἵππους,

---

1 εὖ post ἔφη M ἔφη om. O ἀλλ': ἢ γὰρ O || 2 ante τοῦ add. τὴν U post αἰτίην add. μέχρις ἂν μάθῃς b κρίσσον U || 3 ἀντιφροντισάμενος O ἀποίσῃ bO || 4 ἑαυτὸν O ἀνθ' ὧν: ἀληθῶς U post ἴσως add. δὲ U || 5 ὅσην σπούδην Ub οἵην σπούδην O || 6 πράσσουσι καὶ εἰς τὰ μηδενὸς ἄξια U post βίον add. ἀχρήστως bO || 7 Λέγε φημί: λέγε ἔφην U λέγω O φημὶ λέγε MU || 8 διαλανθάνῃ UV πᾶς: ἅπας MU νοσέων ante πᾶς UbO ὁ ante πᾶς b καὶ om. U οὐκ: οὐδὲ UbO || 9 ἂν om. a γὰρ: δὲ O || 13 ἴθι b δὲ νῦν: τοίνυν O || 15 τρανὸν: τρηχὺ O || 16 φλαῦρα bO γέλωτα ἀνθρώπου MU γελῶ τὰ ἀνθρώπου U μὲν om. MV || 17 κενεᾶ U κενὸν O ἐπιβουλῇσιν b ἐπιβουλαῖσιν U || 18 ἀλγέοντα: ἀνύοντα O ante μόχθους add. πόνους καὶ b^2 || 19 ἀκροτάτους μόχθους καὶ μυχοὺς U χυμους M (et in marg. γρ. καὶ μυχοὺς) ἀμετρίης ἐπιθυμίῃ O ἀμετροίησι b (ante corr.) τήκοντα: τείνοντα U || 20 θορυβευόμενος VM^2 || 21 αὐτὸς om. V ἐλάσσω M (corr. M^2) ante γένηται add. μὴ b οὐδὲ: οὐδὲν O om. U || 22 ante γῆς add. τῆς U δεσμίον U ὧν: ὤν V || 23 ὑπὸ σομφῆς: ἐπισομφῆς MU ἐπιπιπτούσης MUO || 23-4 πολλῷ χρόνῳ ταύτην ἄγοντες (ἔχοντες c) O || 24 ἔχοντες τὴν om. V ἐν om. a καταμένουσιν Ob^2 ἀργύριον MUb || 25 χρύσιον Ub μαστεύοντες om. MU ψήγματα: ῥήγματα καὶ ῥήγματα (sic) V ψήματα M (corr. M^2) ἐγείροντες UM^2 || 26 τῆς: τὰς b om. O || 28 πόδε μίην MV μίην U πολεμίην bO τὸ δὲ μίην Diels Putz. || 29 θαυμάζουσι καὶ πατ. bO || 30 ante τὴν add. καὶ O post τὴν add. δὲ U ὑβρίζουσι O

"Right you are, Hippocrates, but you are as yet unaware of the cause of my laughter. And when you learn it, I am certain that you will take on a better cargo than you brought on your embassy, my laughter, and carry it back as therapy for your country and yourself, and you will be able to instruct all others in virtue. And perhaps in return you will teach me medicine, when you know how passionately people in general, striving for what is not worth striving for, pour out their lives on activities that are of no value, busying themselves with things that deserve laughter." And I said, "Speak, by the gods! Maybe, without it being apparent, the whole world is sick and has no place to send an embassy for therapy. For what could there be outside itself?" And he answered, "There are many infinities of worlds, Hippocrates, and never, my friend, belittle the riches of nature." I said, "But you will teach me that in its own season. I am wary that you will start to laugh even while going through infinity. Know that now you are about to give an explanation of your laughter to the life that we know."

5. He looked straight at me and spoke very clearly: "You think that there are two causes for my laughter, good things and bad. But I laugh at one thing, humanity, brimming with ignorance, void of right action, childish in all aspirations, agonizing through useless woes for no benefit, traveling to the ends of the earth and her boundless depths with unmeasured desire, melting gold and silver, never stopping this acquisitiveness of theirs, ever in an uproar for more, so that they themselves can be less. They have no shame at being called happy for digging gaping holes in the earth using the hands of chained men, some of whom have died from the collapse of porous earth, and others of whom stay on in endless bondage, as though punishment is their native place. They search for gold and silver, seeking out tracks and scrapings of dust, gathering sand from here and there and excising earth's veins for profit, ever turning mother earth into lumps. But it is one and the same earth that they walk on in wonder. Hilarious! They love the laborious, hidden earth as they violate the earth they see. They buy

οἱ δὲ χώρην πολλὴν περιορίζοντες ἰδίην ἐπιγράφουσιν καὶ πολλῆς ἐθέλοντες δεσπόζειν οὐδὲ αὐτῶν δύνανται. γαμεῖν σπεύδουσιν, ἃς μετ' ὀλίγον ἐκβάλλουσιν· ἐρῶσιν, εἶτα μισοῦσι· μετ' ἐπιθυμίης γεννῶσιν, εἶτ' ἐκβάλλουσι τελείους· τίς ἡ κενὴ σπουδὴ καὶ ἀλόγιστος μηδὲν μανίης διαφέρουσα; πολεμοῦσιν ἔμφυλον, ἠρεμίην οὐχ αἱρετίζοντες, ἀντενεδρεύουσι, βασιλέας ἀνδροφονοῦσι· γῆν ὀρύσσοντες ἀργύριον ζητοῦσι, ἀργύριον εὑρόντες γῆν ἐθέλουσι πρίασθαι, ὠνησάμενοι γῆν καρποὺς πιπράσκουσι, καρποὺς ἀποδόμενοι πάλιν ἀργύριον λαμβάνουσι· ἐν ὅσῃσι μεταβολῇσίν εἰσιν, ἐν ὅσῃ κακίῃ. οὐσίην μὴ ἔχοντες οὐσίην ποθέουσι, ἔχοντες κρύπτουσιν, ἀφανίζουσι. καταγελῶ ἐφ' οἷσι κακοπραγέουσιν,
364 ἐπιτείνω τὸν γέλωτα ἐφ' οἷσι δυστυχοῦσι· θεσμοὺς γὰρ ἀλη|θείης παραβεβήκασι φιλονικέοντες ἔχθρην πρὸς ἀλλήλους. δῆριν ἔχουσι μετὰ ἀδελφῶν καὶ τοκήων καὶ πολιτῶν καὶ ταῦτα ὑπὲρ τοιούτων κτημάτων ὧν οὐδεὶς θανὼν δεσπότης ἐστίν. ἀλληλοκτονέουσι, ἀθεσμόβια φρονεῦντες φίλων καὶ πατρίδων ἀπορίην ὑπερορῶσι. πλουτίζουσι τὰ ἀνάξια καὶ τὰ ἄψυχα, ὅλης τῆς οὐσίης ἀνδριάντας ὠνέονται, ὅτι δοκεῖ λαλεῖν τὸ ἄγαλμα· τοὺς δὲ ἀληθέως λαλέοντας μισεῦσι· τῶν γὰρ μὴ ῥηϊδίων ἐφίενται. καὶ γὰρ ἤπειρον οἰκεῦντες θάλασσαν ποθέουσι· καὶ πάλιν ἐν νήσοισιν ἐόντες ἠπείρων γλίχονται· καὶ πάντα διαστρέφουσιν ἐς ἰδίην ἐπιθυμίην. καὶ δοκέουσι μὲν ἐν πολέμῳ ἀνδρείην ἐπαινεῖσθαι, νικῶνται δὲ καθ' ἡμέρην ὑπὸ τῆς ἀσελγείης, ὑπὸ φιλαργυρίης, ὑπὸ τῶν παθέων πάντων ἃ νοσέουσι. Θερσῖται δ' εἰσὶ τοῦ βίου πάντες. τί δὲ τὸν ἐμόν, Ἱππόκρατες, ἐμέμψω γέλωτα; οὐ γὰρ αὐτοὶ τῆς ἰδίης ἀνοίης, ἀλλὰ ἄλλος ἄλλου καταγελῆτε, οἱ μὲν τῶν μεθυόντων, ὅταν αὐτοὶ δοκέωσι νήφειν, οἱ δὲ τῶν ἐρώντων, χαλεπωτέρην νοῦσον νοσεῦντες αὐτοί, οἱ δὲ τῶν πλεόντων, ἄλλοι δὲ τῶν περὶ γεωργίην ἀσχοληθέντων· οὐ συμφωνέουσι γὰρ οὔτε τῇσι τέχνῃσιν οὔτε τοῖσιν ἔργοισιν.

6. Ἐγὼ δέ, Ταῦτα μέν, ἔφην, κρήγυα, Δημόκριτε, οὐδ' ἄλλος τις ἂν εἴη λόγος ἁρμοδιώτερος ἐξαγγέλλων ταλαιπωρίην θνητῶν. ἀλλ' αἱ πρήξιες νομοθετοῦσι τὴν ἀναγκαίην οἰκονομίης τε εἵνεκα καὶ ναυπηγίης καὶ τῆς
366 ἑτέρης πολιτείης, ἐν ᾗ χρεὼν εἶναι τὸν ἄνθρωπον. | οὐ γὰρ ἐς ἀργίην αὐτὸν ἡ φύσις ἐγέννα. ἐκ τούτων δὲ πάλιν φιλοδοξίη χυθεῖσα ἔσφηλε

---

1 post χώρην add. μάλα b πάνυ b^2 πολλῶν bO || 2 ἐθέλουσι V || 3 ἐκβεβλήκασιν UO γεννῶσιν: τεκνοῦσιν O || 4 τελείως O in marg. b: γρ. τίς ἡ κενοσπουδίη καὶ ὁ λογισμὸς || 5 ἔμφυλα O αἱρετίζουσιν UOb (corr. b^2) || 6 ὀρύσσουσιν U ἄργυρον O || 7 ἄργυρον O || 8 πιπρήσκουσι Vb ἀποδεχόμενοι U μεταλαμβάνουσιν O || 9 ἐν om. bO ἐν ὅσοι U post κακίῃ add. πολιτείης O οὐσιην[1] om. Ob (add. b^2) || 10 ante ἀφανιζ. add. ᾗ b καταγελῶ om. O || 12 δηρὴν V δηρὸν b post μετὰ add. δὲ MV || 13 πολιητῶν b || 14 οὐδὲ εἷς VO ἄθεσμα βία φονεύοντες O φονεῦντες corr. in φρονεῦντες M || 15 πατέρων Ub (corr. b^2) || 16 ἀνδριάντα U || 17 λέγοντας UO γὰρ om. O ἰδίων O || 18 ante θαλ. add. κάρτα b || 19 ἤπειρον M -ων V || 20 ἐπαινέσαι O || 22 ἃ om MV νοσεύει V ἂν νοσοῦσι U || 23 αὐτὸς M et in marg. γρ. καὶ αὐτοὶ ἀνοίης: ἂν ὀπῆς V || 24 καταγελῆται b (corr. b^2) καταγελῇ V καταγελᾶ O δοκέουσι M || 25 χαλεπωτέρων U post χαλ. add. ἑτέρην b νοῦσον om. O || 29 αἱ om. M || 29-30 ἀλλὰ πράξεις νομοθ. εἶναι ἀναγκαίας U || 30 οἰκοδομίας U οἰκοδομῆς b (corr. b^2) || 32 φιλοδοξίη b

dogs, they buy horses, they put boundaries around large tracts and claim them for their own: they want to be master of much, and cannot master themselves. They rush to marry women whom they cast out shortly later. They love, then they hate. They beget children in desire, then they cast them out when they are grown. What is this empty and irrational passion, no different from madness? They war on their own kind and do not choose peace, they ambush each other, they murder kings. They dig up the earth in search of silver, and if they find silver they want to buy earth. Having bought earth they sell its fruits and disposing of its fruits they get silver once more. How they vacillate! In what ugliness! When they have no wealth they desire wealth, when they have it they conceal it, make it disappear. I laugh at the things in which they fail, I laugh long at their misfortunes, for they have transgressed the decrees of truth, trying to outdo one another in hatred. They battle with siblings and parents and fellow citizens, and do it for the sort of possessions that no one controls when he is dead. They murder one another, they long for life without restraints while they ignore the helplessness of friends and country. They turn the worthless and the lifeless into wealth; with their whole substance they purchase statues, 'because the pretty statue seems to speak.' But they hate men that actually speak. For they aim at the recherché. If they live on the mainland, they want the sea. If they live on islands they long for mainlands, and twist everything to their own singular desire. In war they seem to approve courage, but they are bested daily by lust, by greed, by all the passions they are sick with. Each one is a Thersites of life. Why did you criticize my laughter, Hippocrates? You people do not laugh at your own stupidity but each laughs at another's, some at drunk people, thinking themselves sober, some at lovers, though they have a worse disease themselves, some at sailors and some at those who practice farming. For they do not have a harmonious relation to the crafts or to useful work."

6. I said, "That is all very agreeable, Democritus, and no other account could describe so fittingly human wretchedness. But activities legislate the wretchedness that is necessary, in running a house, shipbuilding, or public activity in general, which men must be involved in, since nature did not beget them for inactivity. And flowing out of these activities desire to be outstanding has confused and tripped up many people's otherwise right thinking souls, as they

πολλῶν ὀρθογνώμονα ψυχήν, σπουδαζόντων μὲν ἅπαντα ὡς ἐπὶ ἀδιαπτωσίῃ, μὴ κατευτονούντων δὲ τὴν ἀδηλότητα προορᾶσθαι. ἧπου γὰρ τίς, ὦ Δημόκριτε, γαμέων ἢ χωρισμὸν ἢ θάνατον προσεδόκησε; τίς δ' ὁμοίως παιδοτροφέων ἀπώλειαν; ἀλλ' οὐδ' ἐν γεωργίῃ καὶ πλοίῳ καὶ βασιλείῃ καὶ ἡγεμονίῃ καὶ πάνθ' ὅσα ὑπάρχει κατὰ τὸν αἰῶνα. οὐδεὶς γὰρ προὔλαβεν πταῖσαι, ἀλλ' ἀγαθῇσιν ἕκαστος τούτων ἐλπίσι φέρβεται, τῶν δὲ χερειόνων οὐδὲ μέμνηται. μήποτ' οὖν ὁ σὸς γέλως τούτοισιν ἀνάρμοστος;

7. Ὁ δὲ Δημόκριτος, Μάλα, ἔφη, νωθὴς τὸν νόον ὑπάρχεις καὶ μακρὰν γε τῆς ἐμῆς γνώμης ἀπόδημος, Ἱππόκρατες, ἀταραξίης καὶ ταραχῆς μέτρα μὴ ἐπισκοπέων δι' ἄγνοιαν. ταῦτα γὰρ αὐτὰ διανοίῃ φρενήρει διοικέοντες αὐτοί τε ῥηϊδίως ἀπήλλασσον καὶ τὸν ἐμὸν ἐλώφεον γέλωτα· νῦν δ' ὡς ἐπαρηρόσι τοῖσιν ἐν τῷ βίῳ φρενοβλαβεῖς τετύφωνται ἀσυλλογίστῳ διανοίῃ τῆς ἀτάκτου φορῆς, δυσδίδακτοι. νουθεσίη γὰρ αὐτάρκης ὑπῆρχεν ἡ τῶν ξυμπάντων μεταβολὴ ὀξείῃσι τροπῇσι ἐμπίπτουσα, αἰφνίδιον τροχηλασίην παντοίην ἐννοέουσα. οἱ δ' ὡς ἐπαρηρυίῃ καὶ βεβαίῃ ἐκλελησμένοι παθέων κατὰ τὸ ξυνεχὲς συμπιπτόντων ἄλλοτε ἄλλως ποθεῦντες τὰ λυπέοντα, διζήμενοι τὰ μὴ ξυμφέροντα ἐναλινδεῦνται πολλῇσι ξυμφορῇσιν. εἰ δ' ἐμερμήριζεν κατὰ
368 δύναμιν ἰδίην | τὰ ξύμπαντα ἔρδειν, ἀδιάπτωτον ἐφρούρει ζωὴν ἑωυτὸν ἐξεπιστάμενος καὶ ξύγκρισιν ἰδίην σαφῶς κατανοήσας καὶ μὴ τῆς ἐπιθυμίης τὴν σπουδὴν ἀόριστον ἐκτείνων, τὴν δὲ πλουσίην φύσιν καὶ πάντων τιθηνὸν δι' αὐταρκείης ὁρέων. καθάπερ δὲ τῶν παθέων εὐεξίη κίνδυνος πρόδηλος, οὕτως τὸ μέγεθος τῶν εὐτυχημάτων σφαλερόν ἐστι, ἀρίσημοι δ' ἐπὶ τῇσι κακοδαιμονίῃσι ξυνθεωρεῦνται. ἄλλοι δὲ τὰ τῶν πέλας μὴ ἱστορέοντες ὑπὸ τῆς ἰδίης κακοπραγίης ἀπώλοντο, τὰ δῆλα καθάπερ ἄδηλα μὴ θεωρεῦντες, ὑπόδειγμα τὸν μακρὸν βίον ἔχοντες γενομένων καὶ γινομένων, ἐξ ὧν καὶ τὸ ἐσόμενον ἐχρῆν κατανοῆσαι. ταῦθ' ὁ ἐμὸς γέλως· ἄφρονες ἄνθρωποι, πονηρίης δίκας ἐκτίνοντες, φιλαργυρίης, ἀπληστίης, ἔχθρης, ἐνέδρης, ἐπιβουλίης, βασκανίης· ἀργαλέον ἐξειπεῖν πολυμηχανίην κακῶν, ἀπειρίη γάρ τις ἐστὶ κἀν τούτοισι· δολοπλοκίῃσι ἀνθαμιλλεῦντες, σκολιόφρονες, ἀρετῆς δὲ παρ' αὐτοῖσι τρόπος

---

2 ἀδιαπτωσίην O ἀδιάπτωσιν U ἐπὶ διάπτωσιν MV μὴ: ἡμὴ M μηκέτ' εὐτονεόντων O προορίσασθαι O ποῦ O || 3 τίς: τοι a ἢ[1] om. b || 4 ἀπώλειαν ante παιδοτ. U πλοίῳ: πάθω V πλοφ καὶ ναυτιλίῃ O || 5 οὐδὲ εἷς UVO || 6 προὐπέλαβε b προσέλαβε O || 7 ante γε add δέ O οὐδὲ: οὐ O post ἀναρμ. add. ἦ U || 8 νωθὴς ante ἔφη UO || 9 post ἀποδ. add. εἶ b ἰὼν U || 10 μὴ om. O αὐτὰ om. U φρενήρῃ M || 11 τε: δὲ U ante ἀπήλλασον add. ἂν U ἀπηλάσσοντο b(-ττ-)O ἐλώφων U || 12 τοῖσιν: τούτοισιν O τετύφλωνται MU || 14 συμβάντων O || 15 ἐννοέουσα: ἑλίσσουσα UO || 16 ἐκλελησμένη U || 17 ἐμπιπτόντων MU || 18 δ': δέ τις b ἐμερμήριζον U || 19-20 εαυτοῖς ἐξεπιστάμενοι U || 20 κατανοήσαντες U || 21 ἐκτείνοντες U || 22 τιθηνὴν O ὁρέων: ὁδοιπορέων bO ὁδοιποροῦντες U ante εὐεξίῃ add. ἐν O || 23 ἐπισφαλέστερον O || 24 ἐπὶ: ἐν M || 25 ante μὴ add. ὡς M μὴ: δι' U μηδὲν O ἱστορέοντες: θεωρεῦντες Vb in marg. b γρ. παλαιῶν μὴ ἱστορέοντες post τὰ add. δὲ O || 26 καθάπερ ἄδηλα post θεωρ. U ἔχοντες om. V || 27 καὶ γινομένων om. U γινομένων: μὴ γενομένων bO καὶ[II] om. U || 28 ταῦθ' om. U ἐκτείνοντες MUV || 29 ἐνεδρείης O ἐπιβουλῆς UbO || 29-30 ἐργαλέον ὡς εἰπεῖν a || 31 ἀνθομιλλέονται b

strain for everything as though they cannot stumble, for they have not the power to foresee what is hidden. Really, Democritus, who, on marrying, expected separation or death? Similarly, who, in bringing up children foresaw their loss? So also in farming or sailing, or kingship, or leadership, or all the activities of life: nobody ever anticipated failure. Everyone feeds on good hope for those things. Nor is he mindful of the worse possibilities. Isn't your laughter inappropriate for them?"

7. Democritus said, "Your mind is sluggish, Hippocrates. You are far away from my thoughts because in your ignorance you do not look for measures of calm and perturbation.[1] If they managed these things with thoughtful calculation they would easily escape and get relief from my laughter, but as things are, assuming that matters in life are fixed, they are driven crazy by them, deluded by irrational calculation about change that is irregular. They are unteachable. There is inherent instruction in the alteration of all things which falls on them with sharp swerves, which makes us aware of every kind of unanticipated revolution.[2] They, as though it is fixed and secure, forget the sufferings that always befall them, and they desire, time after time, one way and another, things that are a source of grief. In their search for what is inappropriate they tumble about in numerous misfortunes. If one took thought to do everything in accord with his own capacity, he would keep his life erect, he would understand himself and comprehend clearly his own composition, and he would not stretch out boundlessly the eagerness of desire, for he would see that nature is rich and nurses all through her self-sufficiency. And just as blooming health offers clear danger of affections, so is a quantity of good fortune treacherous.[3] Very prominent men are observed to be associated with evil fortune. Other people have been ruined by their own bad luck because they have not looked into what happened to their neighbors. They investigate what is patent just as little as what is obscure, though they have as the example of things that happened and are happening a long life, from which they should figure out what will happen. That is the cause of my laughter. Mindless men who pay the penalty for their baseness, greed, insatiability, enmity, treachery, scheming, malignity. It is painful to relate their various contrivances of evil, for there is an infinity of them too. They try to outdo each other in deviousness, their minds are twisted, their version of

[1] ἀταραξίη and ταραχή, see the note Letter 12, above.

[2] This passage transfers terminology from the motions of atoms to human life.

[3] Democritus alludes here to *Aphorisms* 1.3, "In athletes extremely good condition is treacherous", 'Εν τοῖσι γυμναστικοῖσιν αἱ ἐπ' ἄκρον εὐεξίαι σφαλεραί....

ἐστὶ τὸ χέρειον. φιλοψευδίην γὰρ ἀσκεῦσι, φιληδονίην κοσμέουσι, νόμοισιν ἀπειθεῦντες, ὃ δὲ αὐτῶν κατακρίνει τὴν ἀπροαιρεσίην, μήτε ὁρήσεως μήτε ἀκοῆς μετέχοντες. μούνη δ' αἴσθησις ἀνθρώπου ἀτρεκείῃ διανοίης τηλαυγὴς τό τε ἐὸν καὶ τὸ ἐσόμενον προορεομένη. δυσαρεστεῦνται πᾶσι καὶ πάλιν τοῖσιν αὐτοῖσιν ἐμπελάζονται· ἀρνησάμενοι πλόον πλέουσι, γεωργίην ἀπωσάμενοι αὖτις γεωργοῦσιν· ἐκβάλλοντες γαμετὴν ἑτέρην
370 ἐσάγονται, γεννήσαντες ἔθαψαν, θάψαντες ἐγέννησαν, | πάλιν τρέφουσι· γῆρας ηὔξαντο, ἐς αὐτὸ δ' ἀφικόμενοι στενάζουσι.

8. Ἐν οὐδεμιῇ καταστάσει βεβαίην ἔχουσι τὴν γνώμην· ἡγεμόνες καὶ βασιλεῖς μακαρίζουσι τὸν ἰδιώτην, ὁ δὲ ἰδιώτης ὀρέγεται βασιλείης, ὁ προπολιτευόμενος τὸν χειροτεχνεῦντα ὡς ἀκίνδυνον, ὁ δὲ χειροτέχνης ἐκεῖνον ὡς εὐτονεῦντα κατὰ πάντων. τὴν γὰρ ὀρθὴν κέλευθον τῆς ἠρεμίης οὐ θεωροῦσιν καθαρὴν καὶ λείην καὶ ἀπρόσπταιστον, ἐς ἣν οὐδεὶς τετόλμηκεν ἐμβαίνειν· φέρονται δὲ ἐπὶ τὴν ἀπειθῆ καὶ σκολιὴν τρηχυβατέοντες, καταφερόμενοι καὶ προσκόπτοντες, οἱ δὲ πλεῖστοι ἐκπίπτοντες, ἀσθμαίνοντες ὡς διωκόμενοι, ἐρίζοντες, ὑστερέοντες, προηγεύμενοι. καὶ οὓς μὲν αὐτῶν ἔρωτες ἀτάσθαλοι ὑποπεπρήκασιν ἀλλοτρίης εὐνῆς, φθορῇ, ἀναιδείῃ πισύνους, οὓς δὲ τήκει φιλαργυρίης νοῦσος ἀόριστος. οἱ δ' ἀλλήλοισιν ἀντεπιτίθενται, οἱ δ' ὑπὸ φιλοδοξίης ἐς ἠέρα ἀνενεχθέντες βρίθει κακίης ἐς βυθὸν ἀπωλείης καταφέρονται. κατασκάπτουσι, ἐποικοδομοῦσι· χαρίζονται, εἶτα μετανοοῦσιν ἢ ἀφαιρεῦνται τὰ φιλίης δίκαια, κακοπρηγεῦντες ἐς ἔχθρην τὰ ξυγγενείης πολεμοποιεῦντες, καὶ τούτων πάντων αἰτίη φιλαργυρίη. τί νηπίων ἀθυρόντων διαφέρουσι, παρ' οἷσιν ἄκριτος μὲν ἡ γνώμη, τὸ δὲ προσπεσὸν τερπνόν; ἐν δὲ τοῖσι θυμοῖσι τί περισσὸν ζῴοισιν ἀλόγοισι παραλελοίπασι, πλὴν ὅτι ἐν αὐταρκείῃ μένουσιν οἱ θῆρες; τίς γὰρ λέων ἐς γῆν κατέκρυψε
372 | χρυσόν; τίς ταῦρος πλεονεξίην ἐκορύξατο; τίς πάρδαλις ἀπληστίην κεχώρηκε; διψῇ μὲν ἄγριος σῦς, ὅσον ὕδατος ὠρέχθη, λύκος δὲ δαρδάψας τὸ προσπεσὸν τῆς ἀναγκαίας τροφῆς ἀναπέπαυται. ἡμέρῃσι δὲ καὶ νυξὶ ξυναπτομένῃσιν οὐκ ἔχει θοίνης κόρον ὤνθρωπος· καὶ χρόνων μὲν ἐνιαυσίων τάξις ὀχείης ἀλόγων τέρμα ἐστί· ὁ δὲ τὸ διηνεκὲς οἰστρομανίην ἔχει τῆς ἀσελγείης. Ἱππόκρατες, μὴ γελάσω τὸν κλαίοντα δι' ἔρωτα, ὅτι

---

1 ἀσκεῦσι: ἔχουσι O κάσμου VOb[2] || 2 ὃ: scripsi ὁ mss. ἀπροορισίην b || 3 μετέχοντες: scripsi -ας mss. δ': γὰρ U διανοίῃ MUV || 4 τηλαυγοῦς O || 5 πάλιν post αὐτοῖσιν U || 6 ἀπειπάμενοι b γαμετὴν: deficit hic ms. a || 7 γενν. ἔθαψ. om. O post θαψ. add ἄ. bO || 8 εὔχονται b (corr. b[2]) ante ἐς add. εἶτα O δ' om. bO || 10 ὁ δὲ om. V || 11 πολιτευόμενος UbO δὲ om. O || 13 ἠρεμίης: ἀρετῆς MU οὐδὲ εἷς b || 14 ἐμβῆναι b ἀπειθῆ: μὴ ἀληθῆ U ἐναντίην O || 16 ἀποπίπτοντες b ante ἀσθμαίν. add καὶ. b ὁρίζοντες O || 17 οἷς O ἀτασθάλοις (-λοι d) ὑποπεπτήκασιν O || 18 εὐνῆς, φθορῇ: φώρας εὐνῆς bO ἀναιδείης M φιλαργυρίαν U -ίη O || 20 ἀναχθέντες O ante κακίης add. ὑπὸ b || 21 ἐποικοδομοῦσι: εἶτ' οἰκοδομέουσι b εἶτα οἰκοδομοῦσι U ἐποικοδομοῦντες O | ἢ: καὶ bO, om. U || 23 πολεμοῦσι O κακοποιεῦντες et in marg. γρ. πόλεμον ἐμποιέοντες b πάντων om. O αἴτον O ante φιλαργ. add. ἡ O || 24 ἀθυρώντων MV ἀθυρεόντων bO || 25 θυμοῖσι: μύθοις V || 26 λεόντων O || 27 ante πλεον. add. τὴν b πλεονεξίας ἐκορέσσατο U || 27-8 ἀπληστίην κεχώρηκε: εἰς ἀπληστ. δὲ κεχωρ. U || 28 ὁπόσον U ὠρέχθη: ὀρεχθῇ U κορεσθῇ O || 29 δὲ om. b || 30 θοίνης om. O καὶ om. O || 31 τάξεις U ἀγρίων U ἐστὶ ante τέρμα O τὸ om. V

excellence is superiority in evil. They train themselves in lying, they wear licentiousness as an an ornament, they disobey laws, and, what condemns them to inability to make rational choices, they use neither sight nor hearing. Perception alone is a beacon for right thinking, as it sees what is and foresees what will be. But they are dissatisfied with everything and keep returning to the same things. They renounce sailing, then sail, they reject farming, then farm, they cast off a mate and take another, they beget and bury, and, having buried, beget and rear again. They pray for old age, and if they reach it lament it.

8. There is no condition in which their minds are firm. Kings and leaders call private citizens blessed, the private citizen grasps after a kingdom; the city's leader envies the craftsman as safe, and the craftsman envies the leader as powerful in all things. But they do not see the straight path of tranquility, clear and smooth, which will not make them stumble, but which no one has been bold enough to enter. They are borne along struggling on a treacherous and twisted path, burdened and stumbling; most fall down, panting as though pursued, quarreling, slipping behind, getting ahead. Disgusting loves have set some of them on fire for another's bed as they put their trust in corruption and shamelessness, and some the boundless disease of greed melts away. Some attack one another. Some, carried up into the air by desire for glory, are borne down to the depth of ruin by a burden of evil. They destroy, they build. They give and receive friendship, then they change their minds or withdraw what properly belongs to friendship. When they are in trouble they turn family relations into the enmity of war. Of all this, greed is the cause. How do they differ from children at play, whose minds lack judgment and who take joy in whatever falls to them. In their passions what excess have they left to the irrational beasts, except that beasts retain self-sufficiency? What lion ever hid gold in the ground? What bull butted out of greed? What leopard overfilled himself insatiately? A wild boar feels thirst for as much water as he takes, a wolf devours what he gets for needed nourishment, and stops. But, days and nights strung together, man is never glutted with a banquet. The order of the seasons is a marker for the breeding of dumb beasts, but man perpetually is driven by a gadfly of wantonness. Hippocrates, should I not laugh at a man who weeps for love

ξυμφερόντως ἀποκέκλεισται; μάλιστα δ' ἣν ῥιψοκίνδυνος ἔῃ καὶ φέρηται κατὰ κρημνῶν ἢ βυθῶν πελάγους, ἐπιτενῶ τὸν γέλωτα; μὴ γελάσω τὸν τὴν νῆα πολλοῖσι φορτίοισι βαπτίσαντα, εἶτα μεμφόμενον τῇ θαλάττῃ, ὅτι κατεβύθισεν αὐτὴν πλήρη;

9. Ἐγὼ μὲν οὐδαμῶς δοκέω γελῆν· ἐξευρεῖν δὲ κατ' αὐτῶν ἤθελόν τι λυπηρόν. ἀλλ' οὐδὲ ἰητρικὴν ὑπὲρ τούτων ἐχρῆν εἶναι μητιωμένην παιήονα φάρμακα. ὁ σὸς πρόγονος Ἀσκληπιὸς νουθεσίη σοι γενέσθω· σῴζων ἀνθρώπους κεραυνοῖσιν ηὐχαρίστηται. οὐχ ὁρῇς, ὅτι κἀγὼ τῆς κακίης μοῖρά εἰμι; μανίης διζήμενος αἰτίην ζῷα κατατείνω καὶ ἀνατάμνω, ἐχρῆν δὲ ἐξ ἀνθρώπων τὴν αἰτίην ἐρευνῆσαι. οὐχ ὁρῇς, ὅτι καὶ ὁ κόσμος μισανθρωπίης πεπλήρωται; ἄπειρα κατ' αὐτῶν πάθεα ξυνήθροικε. ὅλος ἄνθρωπος ἐκ γενετῆς νοῦσός ἐστι· τρεφόμενος ἄχρηστος, ἱκέτης βοηθείης· αὐξανόμενος ἀτάσθαλος, ἄφρων διὰ χειρὸς παιδαγωγίης·
374 | θρασὺς ἀκμάζων, παρακμάζων οἰκτρός, τοὺς ἰδίους πόνους ἀλογιστίῃ γεωργήσας· ἐκ μητρῴων γὰρ λύθρων ἐξέθορε τοιοῦτος. διὰ τοῦτο οἱ μὲν θυμικοὶ καὶ ὀργῆς ἀμέτρου γέμοντες, οἱ δ' ἐν φθορῇσι καὶ μοιχείῃσι διὰ παντός, οἱ δ' ἐν μέθῃσι, οἱ δ' ἐν ἐπιθυμίῃσι τῶν ἀλλοτρίων, οἱ δ' ἐν ἀπωλείῃσι τῶν σφετέρων. ὄφελον δύναμις ὑπῆρχεν τὰς ἁπάντων οἰκήσεις ἀνακαλύψαντα μηθ' ἓν ἀφεῖναι τῶν ἐντὸς παρακάλυμμα, εἶθ' οὕτως ὁρᾶν τὰ πρησσόμενα ἔνδον. εἴδομεν ἂν οὓς μὲν ἐσθίοντας, οὓς δὲ ἐμέοντας, ἑτέρους δὲ αἰκίῃσι στρεβλέοντας, τοὺς δὲ φάρμακα κυκέοντας, τοὺς δὲ ξυννοέοντας ἐπιβουλίην, τοὺς δὲ ψηφίζοντας, ἄλλους χαίροντας, τοὺς δὲ κλαίοντας, τοὺς δὲ ἐπὶ κατηγορίην φίλων ξυγγράφοντας, τοὺς δὲ διὰ φιλοδοξίην ἔκφρονας. καί γε τινὲς βαθύτεραι πρήξιες τῶν κατὰ ψυχὴν κευθομένων. καὶ τούτων ὁκόσοι μὲν νέοι, ὁκόσοι δὲ πρεσβῦται, αἰτεῦντες, ἀρνεόμενοι, πενόμενοι, περιουσιάζοντες, λιμῷ θλιβόμενοι, οἱ δὲ ἀσωτίῃ βεβαρημένοι, ῥυπῶντες, δέσμιοι, οἱ δὲ τρυφῇσι γαυριῶντες, τρέφοντες, ἄλλοι σφάττοντες, ἄλλοι θάπτοντες, ὑπερορέοντες ἃ ἔχουσι, πρὸς τὰς

---

1 ῥιψοκινδυνῆ O ἔῃ: ἦν U om. O || 2 βυθῶν ἢ κρημ. O βυθὸν U ante πελάγους add. ἢ V ἐπιτείνω UbM || 3 μεμφόμενον: μεμψάμενον b καὶ μεταμεμφόμενον O || 4 κατεβύθησεν MU αὐτὴν: τὴν bO || 5 οὐδαμῶς: οὖν οὐδ' ἀξίως b οὐκ ἀξίως O || 6 μητιωμένην: Putz. μήτ' ἰωμένην V μήτε ἰωμένην MU μὴ τεχνωμένην bO || 7 παίπονα MV παιώνια O πλείονα U ante ὁ add. καὶ U νουθεσίης M (corr. M^2) || 8 ante σῴζων add. ὁ ἃ U εὐχαριστεῖται bO post ὁρῇς add. δὲ U (hic et in 10) || 8-9 ὅτι τῆς κακίης κἀγὼ μοίρης b ὅτι κἀγὼ τῆς αὐτῆς μοίρης O || 9 ante ζῷα add. καὶ O κατατίνω U κατακτείνω bO || 10 ἐρεύνασθαι U || 11 ante ἄπειρα add. καὶ UbO || 12 συνήθροισεν O ὅλος ὁ ἄνθρ. b || 13 αὐξόμενος UO διὰ χειρὸς: ἐνδεὴς U || 14 post οἰκτρός add. τε. b πόνους: χρόνους O || 15 γεωργῆσαι b ante διὰ add. καὶ b ante οἱ add. καὶ O || 16 νουμικοὶ M ουμικοὶ V ἐν om. M φθορ. καὶ μοιχ.: ξυμφορῇσι καὶ μαχῇσι VM || 17 post παντός add. οὐδ' ἐν μάχαις καὶ ξυμφοραῖς U οἱ... μέθῃσι om. O πιθυμίαις U || 18 ἀπωλείῃ O ὤφελε O || 19 ἀνακαλύψαντας U -αντες b μηδὲν O εἰ δ' et in marg. γρ. εἰθ' U || 20 ὁρᾶν...οὓς δὲ om. V τοὺς μὲν...τοὺς δὲ O ἐσθίονας U || 21 τοὺς... κυκέοντας om. MV κυτοῦντας U ξυνέοντας V || 22 ἐπιβούλην UbO τοὺς^{I}: οὓς b τοὺς^{II}: οὓς bO || 22-3 τοὺς δὲ κλαίοντας om. MV || 23 ἐπὶ κατηγορίῃ ἑων φύλων O ξυγγραφέοντας b τοὺς^{II}: οὓς bO || 24 καί γε τινὲς: καίτοι γε UO καὶ τά γε ἔτι βαθύτερα b || 26 πενόμενοι om. M || 27 βεβολημένοι b (corr. b^2) ῥυπόοντες O || 28 ἄλλοι σφάττοντες om. b anrte θαπτ. add. δὲ O post θαπτ. add. ἄλλοι κλαίοντες U

when it is his good fortune to have been locked out? And especially if man is a daredevil and is carried away down cliffs or in the deeps of the sea, shall I not apply my laugh? And shall I not laugh at the man who lowers his ship in the water with a great cargo and then blames the sea because the sea takes it full to the bottom?

9. I do not think it right to laugh; I wish I could find something to make them grieve. But there should be no medical art contriving healing medicines for them. Let your ancestor Asclepius be your warning. He saved men and got a thunderbolt for thanks. Do you not see that I, too, am a portion of the evil? In looking for the cause of madness I stretch animals out and cut them up, but I should be seeking the cause from men. Don't you see that even the cosmos is full of misanthropy? It has collected an infinity of affections for men. Man as a whole is an illness from birth, while being raised, resourceless, suppliant for aid; as he grows up he is incorrigible, mindless under his teacher's hand; when grown he is reckless, and past his prime he is pitiable, having produced a crop of suffering for himself with irrationality. That is what he is when he leaps forth from his mother's bloody mess. For that reason, some are volatile, brimming with unlimited passion, some live always in corruption and sexual license, some in drink, some in coveting other's goods, some in squandering their own. I wish I had the power to open up everyone's home and leave nothing covering what is within and so see what was being done inside. We would see some people eating, some vomiting, others torturing people with indignities, some mixing poisons, some contriving plots, some voting, some rejoicing, others weeping, some composing accusations against friends, some mad with ambition. And there are deeper actions that are hidden in the soul.[1] And all of them, young and old, are begging, refusing, needy, too well off, pressed by starvation, weighed down by wastefulness, wallowing in filth, chained, proud of their luxuries, some feeding people, others slaughtering them, others burying, people who despise what they

---

[1] Perhaps "There are deeper deeds than those hidden in the soul." This sentence is hardly cogent, and this section generally lacks coherence, but there may be allusion here to an actual statement by Democritus that there is a veritable treasure house of evil hidden within men (Plut. *Animine an corp. aff.* 500 D, Diels-Kranz 68 B 149). κευθομένων is a poetic word which may allude to the often quoted words of Achilles in *Iliad* 9, "I hate like the gates of Hell the man who hides one thing in his heart but says another." ἐχθρὸς γάρ μοι κεῖνος ὁμῶς 'Αΐδαο πύλησιν, ὅς χ' ἕτερον μὲν κεύθῃ ἐνὶ φρεσίν ἄλλο δὲ εἴπῃ.

376 ὑπερορίους κτήσιας ὡρμη|μένοι, οἱ μὲν ἀναίσχυντοι, οἱ δὲ φειδωλοί, οἱ δὲ ἄπληστοι, οἱ μὲν φονεῦντες, οἱ δὲ τυπτόμενοι, οἱ δὲ ὑπερηφανεῦντες, οἱ δὲ ἐπτερωμένοι κενοδοξίῃ· καὶ οἱ μὲν ἵπποισι παρεστῶτες, οἱ δὲ ἀνδράσι, οἱ δὲ κυσίν, οἱ δὲ λίθοισιν ἢ ξύλοισιν, οἱ δὲ χαλκῷ, οἱ δὲ γραφῇσι· καὶ οἱ μὲν ἐν πρεσβείῃσιν, οἱ δ' ἐν στρατηγίῃσιν, οἱ δὲ ἱερωσύνῃσι, οἱ δὲ στεφανηφορίῃσιν· οἱ δὲ ἔνοπλοι, οἱ δὲ ἀποκτεινόμενοι. φέρονται δὲ τούτων ἕκαστοι οἱ μὲν ἐπὶ ναυμαχίην, οἱ δὲ ἐπὶ στρατείην, οἱ δὲ ἐπ' ἀγροικίην, ἕτεροι δὲ ἐπὶ φορτίδας νηῦς, οἱ δὲ ἐς ἀγορήν, ἕτεροι δ' ἐπ' ἐκκλησίην, οἱ δ' ἐπὶ θέητρον, οἱ δὲ ἐς φυγήν, ἄλλοι δὲ ἀλλαχόσε. καὶ οἱ μὲν ἐς φιληδονίην καὶ ἡδυπαθείην καὶ ἀκρασίην, οἱ δὲ ἐς ἀργίην καὶ ῥᾳθυμίην. τὰς ἀναξίους οὖν καὶ δυστήνους σπουδὰς ὀρεῦντες καὶ τοσαύτας, πῶς μὴ χλευάσωμεν τὸν τοιῇσδε ἀκρασίης ἔχοντα βίον αὐτῶν; κάρτα γὰρ ἔλπομαι μηδὲ τὴν σὴν ἰητρικὴν ἀνδάνειν αὐτοῖσιν. δυσαρεστέονται γὰρ ὑπ' ἀκρασίης ἅπασι καὶ μανίην τὴν σοφίην νομίζουσι. ἤπου γὰρ ὑπονοέω λωβᾶσθαί σου τὰ πολλὰ τῆς ἐπιστήμης ἢ διὰ φθόνον ἢ δι' ἀχαριστίην. οἵ τε γὰρ νοσέοντες ἅμα τῷ
378 σῴζεσθαι τὴν | αἰτίην θεοῖσιν ἢ τύχῃ προσνέμουσι, πολλοὶ δὲ τῇ φύσει προσάψαντες. ἐχθαίρουσι τὸν εὐεργετήσαντα, σμικροῦ δεῖν προσαγανακτεῦντες εἰ νομίζονται χρεωφειλέται. οἵ τε πολλοὶ τὸ τῆς ἀτεχνίης ἐφ' ἑωυτοῖσιν ἔχοντες αἴδριες ἐόντες καθαιροῦσι τὸ κρέσσον· ἐν ἀναισθήτοισι γάρ εἰσιν αἱ ψῆφοι. οὔτε δ' οἱ πάσχοντες συνόμιλοι εἶναι θέλουσι οὔτε οἱ ὁμοτεχνεῦντες μαρτυρεῖν. φθόνος γὰρ ἐνίσταται. οὐκ ἀπείρῳ σοὶ τῶν τοιούτων λεσχηνέω ταῦτα, σαφέως δὲ εἰδὼς ταῦτα ἐν ἀναξιοπαθείῃσί σε πολλάκις γεννηθέντα καὶ οὐ δι' οὐσίην ἢ βασκανίην φιλοτωθάσσοντα. ἀτρεκείης γὰρ οὐδεμία οὔτε γνῶσις οὔτε μαρτυρίη.

10. Ἐπεμειδία λέγων ταῦτα καί μοι, Δαμάγητε, θεοειδής τις κατεφαίνετο καὶ τὴν προτέρην αὐτοῦ μορφὴν ἐξελελήσμην καί φημι, Ὦ

---

1 ὑπερορίους: ἐλπίζομένας UbO κτήσιας: πρήξιας O ὡρμήμενοι O || 2 οἱ μὲν φονεῦντες: οἱ μὲν φονεύοντες Ub οἱ δὲ μὴ φρονέοντες O ὑπερηφανεύοντες V ὑπερηφανοῦνται U || 3 ἐπαιρόμενοι UOb^{2} καινοδοξίη M (corr. M^{2}) || 4 ξύλ. ἢ λίθ. U οἱ δὲ χαλ...γραφ. om. bO ἐν om. bO || 5 ἐν om. bO ante ἱερω. add. ἐν UO στεφανηφοροῦντες bO || 6 ἐν ὅπλοισιν O || 7 οἱ δὲ ἐπὶ στρατ. om. MV στρατηγίην O οἱ δὲ ἐπ' ἀγρ. om. U φορτίδας om. UbO || 8 ἕτεροι: οἱ UbO ἐπ': ἐς b || 9 φυγαδείην O -δίην b -δείαν U δὲ om. O καὶ^{1} om. bO || 10 ante δυστ. add. τὰς O || 11 σπουδὰς: σπουδὰς τοιαύτας bO ψυχὰς τοιαύτας U χλευάσωμαι V || 11-12 τοιῇσδε ἀκρασίης: τοιάνδε ἀκρασίαν U ἀκρασίην bO || 13 ἀνδάνη U ὑπ' ἀκρ: ἀκροήσει O αὐτῇ et in marg. γρ. τῇ ἀκροάσει b ἅπασι om. UbO || 14 ἤπου...ὑπον.: ἤκουσα γὰρ ὑπὸ νοσεύντων O λωβᾶσθαί: σαφέως λωβάζεσθαι O ὡς σαφῶς λωβᾶσθαι U σαφέως τωθάζεσθαι b (λωβᾶσθαί σοι b^{2}) || 15 δι' ἀχριστίην M τῷ: τὸ b || 16 ante θεοῖσιν add. ἢ O τῇ φύσει: τῇ ἰδία φύσι U || 17 ἐχθραίνουσι Ob (corr. b^{2}) || 18 νομίζωνται b post χρέωφ. add. εἶναι b τε om. O πολὺ Vb τὸ: τὰ U || 19 ἐφ': ἐν UbO τε post αἴδρ. add. O καθαιροῦσι: ἐχθραίνουσι O || 19-20 ἐν αἰσθητοῖσι O || 20 συνόμιλοι εἶναι: ἐξομολογέειν bO ὁμολογεῖν U || 22 ἀπείρῳ σοι: ἀπείροις U ἄπειρος σὺ bO ἀπείρως οἱ M λεσχηνέω: scripsi λεσχηνέων MV λεσχημάτων U λεσχέων bO || δὲ om. UO ταῦτα^{II} om. UbO || 23 ἀξιοπαθείησι Vb οὐ om. UbO οὐσίην: αἰτίαν U ἢ: τε καὶ O καὶ διὰ U σέο καὶ διὰ b || 24 φιλωτωθάσοντα U φιλοτώθασον bO φῖλον ταθάσοντα V ἀτρεκὴς U οὐδεμιῆς Ob (corr. b^{2}) οὔτε om. bO || 25 post Ἐπεμ. add. δὲ U θεοειδή U τις om. b || 26 καὶ τῆς πρώτης αὐτοῦ μορφῆς ἐκλαθόμενος b ἐκλελησμένην UV ἐκλελήσμην M καί φημι: φημὶ δὲ b

have while pursuing others' possessions, some shameless, others stingy, others insatiable, some murdering, others beaten, others arrogant, others soaring on wings of false pride. Some beside themselves for horses, some for men, some for dogs, some for stones or wood, some for bronze, some for paintings; some men in embassies, others in military command, others in priesthoods, others wearing crowns of victory; and some under arms, some killing; each of these is borne along, towards sea battles, or fighting on land, or farming, or merchant ships, or the market place, the assembly, or the theater, and some into exile, others elsewhere, some to love of pleasure, self-indulgence and wantonness, and some to laziness and indifference. When we see these wretched, unworthy pursuits, so many of them, how can we fail to mock at their life which cleaves to such wantonness. Really, I expect that your medical science is not even pleasing to them. They are disaffected from everything by their wantonness, and they consider wisdom madness. Yes, I suspect that they have slandered most of your learning through jealousy or ingratitude. If they are sick, as soon as they are saved they assign the cause to the gods or to fortune, and many of them fasten the cause on Nature. They hate their benefactor, and they are almost more angry if they think they are indebted. And the majority, void of knowledge or training themselves, in their ignorance destroy what is superior, for the votes belong to the imperceptive. Even those who have experience of it do not want to associate with it, nor fellow practitioners to bear witness to it, for they are full of jealousy. I am not saying this to you because you have no experience of such things; I know well that you have often been put in undeserved positions in regard to these things and that you are not one who mocks people on account of money or from spite. For of strict truth there is neither knowledge nor testimonial."

10. He smiled as he said these things, and to me, Damagetus, he seemed like a divine figure, and I forgot his earlier form. I said, "Oh great Democritus, I shall

Δημόκριτε μεγαλόδοξε, μεγάλας γε πάντων σῶν ξεινίων δωρεὰς ἐς Κῶ ἀποίσομαι· πολλοῦ γάρ με τῆς σοφίης θαυμασμοῦ πεπλήρωκας. ἀπονοστέω
380 δέ σου κῆρυξ ἀληθείην ἀνθρωπίνης φύσεως | ἐξιχνεύσαντος καὶ νοήσαντος, θεραπείην δὲ λαβὼν παρὰ σεῦ τῆς ἐμῆς διανοίης ἀπαλλάσσομαι τῆς ὥρης τοῦτο ἀπαιτούσης καὶ τῆς τοῦ σώματος τημελείης. αὔριον δὲ καὶ κατὰ τὸ ἑξῆς ἐν ταὐτῷ γενησόμεθα. ἀνιστάμην ταῦτα εἰπὼν καὶ ὃς ἦν ἕτοιμος ἀκολουθεῖν. προσελθόντι δέ τινι οὐκ οἶδ' ὅθεν ἐπεδίδου τὰ βιβλία. κἀγὼ ξυντονώτερον ἤπειξα καὶ πρὸς τοὺς ἐόντως Ἀβδηρίτας ἐπὶ τῇ σκοπιῇ ἀναμένοντάς με· Ἄνδρες, ἔφην, τῆς πρὸς ἐμὲ πρεσβείης χάρις ὑμῖν πολλή. Δημόκριτον γὰρ εἶδον, ἄνδρα σοφώτατον, σωφρονίζειν ἀνθρώπους μοῦνον δυνατώτατον. ταῦτ' ἔχω σοι περὶ Δημοκρίτεω, Δαμάγητε, φράζειν γηθόσυνα πάνυ. ἔρρωσο.

18. Δημόκριτος Ἱπποκράτει εὖ πράττειν.

Ἐπῆλθες ἡμῖν ὡς μεμηνόσιν, ὦ Ἱππόκρατες, ἐλλέβορον δώσων πεισθεὶς ἀνοήτοισιν ἀνδράσι, παρ' οἷσιν ὁ πόνος μανίη ἐκρίνετο. ἐτυγχάνομεν δὲ περὶ κόσμου διαθέσεως καὶ πολογραφίης ἔτι τε ἄστρων οὐρανίων ξυγγράφοντες. γνοὺς δὲ τὴν ἐπὶ τούτοισι φύσιν ὡς ἀκεραίως κάρτα ἐπιδεδημιουργημένα καὶ ὡς τηλοῦ μανίης καὶ παραφρονήσεως καθέστηκεν, ἐμεῖο μὲν φύσιν ἐπῄνεσας, ἀπηνέας δὲ καὶ μεμηνότας κείνους ἔκρινας. ὁκόσα γὰρ ἰνδαλμοῖσι διαλλάττοντα ἀνὰ τὸν ἠέρα πλάζει
382 ἡμέας, ἃ δὴ κόσμῳ ξυνορᾶται | καὶ ἀμειψιρυσμέοντα τέτευχε, ταῦτα νόος ἐμὸς φύσιν ἐρευνήσας ἀτρεκέως ἐς φάος ἤγαγε· μάρτυρες δὲ τούτων βίβλοι ὑπ' ἐμεῖο γραφεῖσαι. χρὴ οὖν καὶ σέ, ὦ Ἱππόκρατες, μὴ τοιουτοτρόποισιν ἀνδράσι ξυνέρχεσθαι καὶ ξυνομιλεῖν, ὧν νόος ἀκρόπλοος καὶ ἀβέβαιος καθέστηκεν. εἰ γάρ τοι πεισθεὶς ὡς μεμηνότα με ἐπότισας, ἐν πινυτῇ μανίῃ ἂν ἐγεγόνει καὶ σέο τέχνην κατεμέμψαντο ὡς παραιτίην

---

1 μεγαλόξενε O γε: τε MV γὰρ O πάντων: τῶν UbO ‖ 2 ante σοφ. add. σῆς Ub ‖ 3 δέ: τε O ἀληθείης UM (corr. M[2]) post ἀληθ. add. δὲ V φύσιν U post νοήσαντος add. καὶ λαλήσαντος bO ‖ 4 δὲ: τε O παρὰ σοῦ post διανοίας U ‖ 5 ἀπαιτ: ἀξιούσης O ἀπατούσης U ἐπιμελείας U καὶ[II] om. O ‖ 6 ἀνισταμένην U ἕτοιμος ἦν O ‖ 7 ἐπακολουθεῖν bO ὅκοθεν M ὅποθεν b ἀπεδίδου MU ‖ 8 ἐπείξας bO καὶ om. bO ὄντας MUO τῆς σκοπιᾶς U ‖ 9 ὑμῖν om. UbO ‖ 11 δυνάμενον O φράζειν, Δαμ. V ‖ 12 γηθοσύνας U γηθόσυνος bO post πάνυ add. γε b

18. Mss. MUVbO(=cd) 14 ὦ ἱππ. post ἡμῖν bO ‖ 15 πόνος: κόσμος c post πόνος add. τῆς ἀρετῆς MUb κρίνεται MUbO post δὲ add. τότε U ‖ 16 πολυγραφίας U ‖ 17 γνώσῃ M γνώσει U γνωθεὶς b γνῶθι O ἐπὶ τούτοισι: τουτέων bO ἀκεραίως: ἀκαίρως Mb[2] ἀτρεκέως UbO ‖ 18 ἐπιδεδημ.: εἴη δεδημ. UbO ‖ 19 καθεστήκοι bO ἀπηνέας... κείνους: ἄφρονας δὲ ἐκείνους καὶ ἀπηνεῖς καὶ μεμηνότας U ‖ 20 διαλλάττονται U ‖ 21 κόσμος U συνεορᾶται b ἀμειψιροῖς μιῆς ἐόντα M ἀψιμόροις μιησέοντα V ἀμαψιροισμιη ἐόντα et in marg. γρ. καὶ ἀμειψιρυσίημιν b ἄμεινον U ἀμαψιροῖς μιῆς (μιῇ c) ἐόντα O corr. Li. ταῦτα: τούτων U ‖ 23 τοιούτοις τρόποις U ‖ 24 ἀκρόπαθος V ἀκρόπολις UM ‖ 25 τοι om. O post πεισθεὶς add. τούτοισ(ιν) UbO ἐν πιν.: ἡ πινυτὴ b ἡ πιτύνη O ‖ 26 μανίῃ M ἂν om. V ἐγεγόνειν MV ἐγεγόνη U τέχνης U ante κατέμεμψ. add. ἂν UbO ὡς παραιτίην: ὥσπερ αἴτιον b (-ίην b[2]) ὡς παραίτιον O

carry the great gifts of all your friendship back to Cos. You have filled me with great wonder at your wisdom. I shall go away as herald that you have tracked down and understood the truth of human nature. And taking from you the therapy for my intellect I shall go away since the hour and the tendance of the body demand it. But tomorrow and the day after we shall be in the same place." I said that and rose, and he was ready to go with me. Someone came forward from somewhere, and he gave his book-rolls to him. I went off quickly to the genuine Abderites who were waiting for me at their lookout. I said, "Men, many thanks for your embassy to me. For I have seen Democritus, wisest of men, alone most capable of teaching mankind virtue."

That is what I have to tell you about Democritus, Damagetus. Happy news indeed! Be well!

18. Democritus to Hippocrates. Greetings.

You came to me to administer hellebore, on the assumption that I was mad, persuaded by mindless men in whose judgment my labor was madness. As it happened, I was writing about the disposition of the cosmos, about the heavens and about the stars. Since you know the nature that is in those things, with what purity they are ordered, and how far from madness and delirium they are, you praised my nature and judged those people crude and insane. All those things that go through the air and confuse us by altering their appearances, things which are seen in the universe and which change their forms, all these has my intellect brought unerringly to light, searching out their nature, as my books about those things bear witness.[1] Hippocrates, you should not have associated with men of such character, whose intellects are superficial and infirm. If you had given me the drink, as being mad, madness would have come in that drink, and they would

---

[1] This letter seems to refer to titles of works by Democritus: περὶ κόσμου, "On the Universe", πολογραφία, "Description of the Heavens", περὶ ἀστρονομίας, "On Study of the Stars", περὶ τῶν διαφερόντων ῥυσμῶν, "On Varieties of Configuration", and περὶ ἀμειψιρυσμίων, "On Changes of Configuration". Democritus used the verb ἀμειψιρυσμεῖν, apparently, to describe changes of form, and the noun σκῆνος for body ("structure") as opposed to soul. See D-K, *Vorsokr*. 68 C 5, B 57, 270 etc.

παρακοπῆς γεγενημένην. ἐλλέβορος γὰρ ὑγιαίνουσι μὲν δοθεὶς ἐπισκοτεῖ διάνοιαν, μεμηνόσι δὲ κάρτα ὠφελεῖν εἴωθεν. ἐννοήθητι γάρ· εἰ μὴ κατειλήφεις με γράφοντα, ἀνακεκλιμένον δὲ ἢ σχέδην περιπατοῦντα καὶ προσομιλέοντα ἐμαυτῷ ὁτὲ μὲν δυσχεραίνοντα, ὁτὲ δὲ μειδιῶντα ἐπὶ τοῖσιν ἐννοουμένοισιν ὑπ' ἐμεῖο καὶ τοῖσι μὲν προσομιλέουσι τῶν γνωρίμων οὐ προσέχοντα, ἐφιστάντα δὲ τὴν διάνοιαν καὶ σκεπτόμενον ἐκπάγλως, ᾠήθης ἂν Δημόκριτον κατά γε ὄψιος κρίσιν ἐκ τῶν ὁρεομένων μανίης εἰκόνι ἐοικέναι. χρὴ οὖν τὸν ἰητρὸν μὴ μόνον ὄψει τὰ πάθη κρίνειν, ἀλλὰ καὶ πρήγματι τούς τε ῥυθμοὺς ἀνακρίνειν ὡς ἐπὶ τὸ πλεῖστον, καὶ πότερον ἄρχοιτο τὸ πάθος ἢ μεσάζοι ἢ λήγοι, καὶ διαφορὴν καὶ ὥρην καὶ ἡλικίην
384 παρατηροῦντα ἰητρεύειν τὸ πάθος οὐλομελίην τε τοῦ | σκήνεος. ἐκ γὰρ τούτων ἁπάντων εὐχερῶς τὴν νοῦσον εὑρήσεις. ἀπέσταλκα δέ σοι τὸν περὶ μανίης λόγον. ἔρρωσο.

19. Τὸν περὶ μανίης λόγον αὐτῷ γραφέντα ἐν τῷ Περὶ ἱερῆς νούσου.

Μαινομένῳ δέ, ὡς ἔφην ἐν τῷ Περὶ ἱερῆς νούσου, ὑπὸ ὑγρότητος τοῦ ἐγκεφάλου, ἐν ᾧ ἐστι τὰ τῆς ψυχῆς ἔργα, ὅταν ὑγρότερος τῆς φύσιος ᾖ ἀνάγκη κινεῖσθαι, κινουμένου δὲ μήτε τὴν ὄψιν ἀτρεμίζειν μήτε τὴν ἀκοήν, ἀλλὰ ἄλλοτε ἄλλα ὁρᾶν τε καὶ ἀκούειν, τήν τε γλῶσσαν τοιαῦτα διαλέγεσθαι οἷα ἂν βλέπῃ τε καὶ ἀκούῃ ἑκάστοτε. ὅσον δὲ ἂν ἀτρεμίσῃ ὁ ἐγκέφαλος, τοσοῦτον καὶ φρονεῖ χρόνον ὁ ἄνθρωπος. γίνεται δὲ ἡ διαφθορὰ τοῦ ἐγκεφάλου ὑπὸ φλέγματος καὶ χολῆς. γνώσῃ δὲ ἑκάτερα ὧδε· οἱ μὲν γὰρ ὑπὸ φλέγματος μαινόμενοι ἥσυχοί τε εἰσὶ καὶ οὐ βοηταὶ οὐδὲ θορυβώδεις, οἱ δὲ ὑπὸ χολῆς πρῆκται καὶ κακοῦργοι καὶ οὐκ ἠρεμαῖοι. ἢν μὲν ξυνεχῶς μαίνωνται, αὗται αἱ προφάσιές εἰσιν, ἢν δὲ δείματα καὶ φόβοι, ὑπὸ μεταστάσιος γίνεται τοῦ ἐγκεφάλου θερμαινομένου ὑπὸ χολῆς ὁρμώσης ἐπ' αὐτὸν κατὰ τὰς φλέβας τὰς αἱματίτιδας, ὅταν δὲ ἀπέλθῃ ἡ χολὴ πάλιν ἐς τὰς φλέβας καὶ τὸ σῶμα πέπαυται. ἀνιῆται δὲ καὶ ἀσῆται καὶ ἐπιλήθεται παρὰ καιρὸν ψυχομένου τοῦ ἐγκεφάλου ὑπὸ φλέγματος, καὶ ξυνισταμένου παρὰ τὸ ἔθος. ὅταν δὲ ἐξαπίνης ὁ ἐγκέφαλος διαθερμαίνηται ὑπὸ χολῆς κατὰ τὰς φλέβας τὰς εἰρημένας

---

1 γενόμενον b (-ην b[2]) μὲν om. V ‖ 2 μεμηνότας V post δὲ add. δοθεὶς bO ὠφελεῖ O εἴωθεν om. O ἐννοήθητι: Putz. ᾠήθην MV νωθῆτε U τί b γνῶθι O post γάρ add. ὡς O ‖ 3 καταλελαβήκεις O ἀνακεκλλιμένον δὲ: ἀλλ' ἀνακεκ. O ἀνακείμενον δὲ Mb σχεδὸν MV σχολῇ U ‖ 4 ἐμαυτῷ: ἑαυτῷ U ἑαυτῷ καὶ πολλάκις bO ποτὲ...ποτὲ U ὅτε...ὅδε M ‖ 5 τῶν γνωρίμων om. U ‖ 6 ἐφιστάνοντα bO ἐφιστάντε U ἐφίστανται V ἐκπάγλως: ἱκανῶς UbO ‖ 7 ᾠήθης: ἔγνως bO in marg. γρ. ἐκπάγλως ᾠήθης b γε: τὴν O ‖ 8 χρὴ οὖν: τοιοῦτον οὖν χρὴ b μόνον: μόνῃ τῇ V ‖ 9 πρήγμασιν b πράγμασι O ῥυθμοὺς: ἐρευγμοὺς Ob (corr.b[2]) ‖ 10 μεσάζει U post ἡλικ. add. καὶ MV post ἡλικ. b habet spatium ex erasura ‖ 11 παρατηροῦντα: παρατηρέειν εἶτα Ob (corr.b[2]) οὐλομελίην τε: οὔτε μετὰ τὴν μελέτην U ‖ 12 τὴν...εὑρήσεις: ἂν τὰς νούσους εὕροις (εὑρήσεις O) bO ἀπέστειλα bO

19. Mss. MUVbc 14 ante τὸν add. ὁ περὶ μανίης λόγος MU Δημόκριτος Ἱπποκράτει περὶ μανίας (om. τὸν...νούσου) b ‖ 15 Μαινομένῳ...νούσου om. V ὑγροτέρας U ‖ 16 ᾖ: ἔστιν b ‖ 17 τὴν[II] om. U ‖ 18 ἄλλοτε: ἄλλο τι U ἄλλα ὁρᾶν: *Morb. sac.* ἀλλοίην Vbc ἀλλοίειν U ἀλλοῖ ἦν M ‖ 19 βλέπει U ἀκούει U ‖ 26 τὰς[I] om. MU ἡ om. U ‖ 27 πέπαυνται bc ‖ 28 post ἐγκεφάλου add. et iterum del. θερμαινομένου ὑπὸ χολῆς ὁρμώσης V ‖ 30 προειρημένας bc

have blamed your science as contributing to insanity. Hellebore given to the healthy darkens the mind, but it generally helps the mad. Consider, if you had found me not writing, but reclining, or walking around slowly, communing with myself, sometimes exasperated, sometimes smiling at my inner thoughts, not attending to conversation of acquaintances, but with my mind entirely engaged in intense investigation, you would have thought that Democritus, by the eye's judgment from things seen, was the image of madness. The physician must judge affections not by the eye only, but from their action infer the configurations insofar as he can, and whether the affection is at its beginning, or middle, or is departing; making close observation of peculiarity, season and age, he should treat the affection and the totality of the structure. For, from all these things you will readily discover the disease. I have sent you my treatise on insanity. Be well!

19. The discourse on madness written by him in *Sacred Disease*.[1]

When a person, as I said in *Sacred Disease*, is mad from moisture in the brain, where the functions of the soul reside, whenever his brain is wetter than is natural, of necessity it is put in motion, and when it is in motion neither sight nor hearing is steady, a person sees and hears now one thing, now another, and his speech says whatever he is seeing or hearing at each moment. So long as the brain is steady, a person is sane. But corruption of the brain comes from bile and phlegm. You will recognize the two kinds as follows: those who are mad because of phlegm are quiet, not loud or disruptive, but those mad from bile are violent, troublesome, are not calm. For continuous madness these are the causes. But if there are frights and terrors, they come from disturbances of the brain when it is heated by bile rushing into it through the blood vessels. When the bile goes back again into the vessels, and the body they stop. One experiences distress, nausea and amnesia when the brain is chilled inappropriately by phlegm, and is compacted more than usual. And when the brain is suddenly heated by bile in the

[1] The descriptions of madness are excerpts from *Sacred Disease* 17 (Littré 6.388-390) and from *Epidemics* 5.80 and 5.81 (Li. 5.250-252). The original texts do not seem to be perfectly understood by the excerpter. Notable is the use of ὑποστροφαί, "relapses," as a symptom of madness in reference to *Epid.* 5.80. I have translated it "failings."

ἐπιζέσαντος αἵματος, ἐνύπνια ὁρεῦσι φοβερὰ καὶ ὡς ἐγρηγορότι τὸ πρόσωπον φλογιᾷ, καὶ οἱ ὀφθαλμοὶ ἐρυραίνονται, καὶ ἡ γνώμη ἐπινοεῖ τι
386 κακὸν ἐργάζεσθαι. τοῦτο καὶ ἐν τῷ ἐνυπνίῳ | πάσχει. ὅταν δὲ τὸ αἷμα σκεδασθῇ πάλιν ἐς τὰς φλέβας, πέπαυται. ἐν δὲ τῷ πέμπτῳ τῶν Ἐπιδημιῶν ἱστόρησας ᾧ ἐγίνετο ἀφωνίη, ἄγνοια, παραληρήσεις συχναὶ καὶ ὑποστροφαί. ἡ δὲ γλῶσσα σκληρή, καὶ εἰ μὴ διακλύσαιτο, λαλεῖν οὐχ οἷός τε ἦν, καὶ σφόδρα πικρὴ τὰ πολλά. φλεβοτομίη ἔλυσεν, ὑδροποσίη, μελίκρητον, ἐλλεβόρων πόσιες. οὗτος ὀλίγον ἐπιζήσας χρόνον ἐτελεύτησεν. ἄλλος ἦν ὅν, ὅτε ἐς πότον ὁρμῴη, φόβος τῆς αὐλητρίδος ἐλάμβανεν εἰ ἀκούσειεν αὐλούσης. ἡμέρης δὲ ἀκούων οὐδὲν ἔπασχεν.

20. Ἱπποκράτης Δημοκρίτῳ εὖ πράττειν.

Ἰητρικῆς τέχνης, ὦ Δημόκριτε, κατορθώματα μὲν οἱ πολλοὶ τῶν ἀνθρώπων οὐ παντάπασιν ἐπαινοῦσιν, θεοῖσι δὲ πολλάκις προσαρτῶσιν. ἢν δέ τι ἡ φύσις ἀντιπρήξασα ὑπεκλύσῃ τὸν θεραπευόμενον, τότε ἰητρὸν καταμέμφονται παρέντες τὸ θεῖον. καὶ ἔγωγε δοκέω πλείονα μεμψιμοιρίην ἢ τιμὴν κεκληρῶσθαι τὴν τέχνην. ἐγὼ μὲν γὰρ ἰητρικῆς ἐς τέλος οὐκ ἀφῖγμαι καίπερ ἤδη γηραλέος καθεστώς, οὐδὲ γὰρ ὁ τῆσδε εὑρέτης Ἀσκληπιός, ἀλλὰ καὶ αὐτὸς ἐν πολλοῖσι διεφώνησε, καθάπερ ἡμῖν ξυγγραφέων βίβλοι παραδεδώκασιν. ἡ μὲν οὖν ὑπὸ σέο ἐπισταλεῖσα ἡμῖν ἐπιστολὴ κατεμέμφετο περὶ τῆς φαρμακείης τοῦ ἐλλεβόρου. ἐσήχθην μὲν οὖν, ὦ Δημόκριτε, ὡς μεμηνότα ἐλλεβοριῶν, οὐ καταμαντευσάμενος ὅστις ποτ' εἴης. ὡς δ' ἐντυχὼν ἔγνων οὐ μὰ Δία παραφρονήσεως ἔργον, ἀλλὰ σχεδὸν ἀποδοχῆς πάσης, κάρτα σὴν φύσιν ἐπῄνεσα ἄριστόν τε φύσιος ἑρμηνευτὴν καὶ κόσμου ἔκρινα, τοὺς δὲ ἐσαγαγόντας με ἐμεμψάμην ὡς μεμηνότας· φαρμακείης γὰρ αὐτοὶ ἔχρηζον. ἐπειδὴ τοίνυν ταὐτόματον ἡμέας ἐς τὸ αὐτὸ ἤγαγεν, ὀρθῶς ποιήσεις ἐπιστέλλων ἡμῖν πυκνότερον καὶ
388 μεταδιδοὺς τῶν ὑπὸ σέο γραφομένων ξυνταγμά|των. ἀπέσταλκα δέ σοι καὶ αὐτὸς τὸν Περὶ ἐλλεβορισμοῦ λόγον. ἔρρωσο.

---

2 φλόγια bc ἐρεύθονται bc ‖ 3 ὕπνῳ bc ‖ 5 ᾧ: ὡς MUV παραλήρησις MV ‖ 7 ἧ V ‖ 8 τεύτησεν M (corr. M^2) ‖ 9 ὅν: ὅς U om. M ὅτε: ὅτι U ὁρμᾶ ἢ V ὁρηὼν U φόβον U

20. Mss. MUVbO(=cd) 13 πάμπολλοι U ‖ 14 οὐ: οὗτοι U πολλάκις: τὰ πολλὰ U προσάπτουσιν Vb (corr. b^2) ‖ 15 ἀντιπρήξασα: ἀντιπράξῃ καὶ O ὑπεκλύσῃ: ὑποκλύσηται V ἀπολέσῃ M^2bO ἀπολέσει U θεραπεύοντα M τότε: τὸν bO om. M ἰατροὺς U ‖ 16 ἐγώγε: ἐγὼ Ob (corr. b^2) ‖ 17 μεμψιμυρίην M γὰρ om. b (add. b^2) ‖ 18 ἤδη om. Ub (add. b^2) ‖ 19 εὐεργετὴς b (corr. b^2) ἐν πολλοῖσι om. O ‖ 20 οὖν om. V add. altera manus ἀποσταλεῖσα bO ‖ 21 ἐπιστολὴν U περὶ om. O τοῦ ἐλλεβορισμοῦ τῆς φαρμακείας U ‖ 22 ἐλλεβορίσων O ‖ 23 ἔγνων: εἶδον O ‖ 24 σχεδὸν om. U ἀποδοχῆς om. M (add. in marg. M^2) σὴν: τὴν UO lacunam habet b πάσης... λιτι τετριμμένον (infra, p.100 lin. 6) folio uno amisso. ‖ 24-5 ἑρμηνέα φύσιος O ‖ 25 εἰσάγοντάς V ‖ 27 ξυνήγαγεν O ‖ 28 γεγραμμένων O ἀπέστειλα O ‖ 29 post Περὶ add τοῦ. M ἔρρωσο om. O

vessels I mentioned, when the blood has boiled, they see fearful dreams, the face is inflamed as in one who is awake, the eyes grow red, the mind imagines some horrible action. This is experienced even in the dream, but it stops when the blood is distributed again to the vessels. In *Epidemics V* you described a man who experienced voicelessness, and disorientation, frequent delirious talk, failings. His tongue was hard, and if he did not irrigate it he could not speak, and it was generally very bitter. Phlebotomy brought relief, drinking water, honey-water, draughts of hellebore. He, after surviving a short time, died. And there was another who was seized, when he went to a symposium, by terror of the flute girl if he heard her playing. But when he heard it in the daytime he suffered no effect.

20. Hippocrates to Democritus. Do well!

Most people do not praise the successes of medical science, and they often attribute them to the gods. But if nature is recalcitrant and weakens the patient, then they blame the physician and pass over the divine. I think that medical science is allotted more reproach than honor.[1] And, in fact, I myself have not reached the goal of medicine, though I am now old. And indeed, neither did its founder, Asclepius, but he too, was inconsistent in many things, as books of those who recorded it have conveyed to us. The letter sent by you to me offered criticism about treatment with hellebore. I was summoned to give you hellebore on the assumption that you were mad, Democritus, and I had not divined what kind of person you were. But when I met you I knew yours was not the work of madness, but of virtually total control of mind. I praised your nature and judged you an excellent interpreter of Nature and the universe, and I criticized those who had brought me, and called them mad. They needed the medicine, I said. Since chance brought us together, you will do well to write to me often and share your compositions. I have sent you the discourse on hellebore. Be well!

---

[1] Cf. *Diseases 1*.8 (Li. 6.156) and *Law* 1 (Li. 4.638) for the expression of similar sentiments.

21. Περὶ Ἐλλεβορισμοῦ Ἱπποκράτης Δημοκρίτῳ

Τοῖσι μὴ ῥηϊδίως ἄνω καθαιρομένοισι πρὸ τῆς πόσιος προϋγραίνειν τὰ σώματα πλείονι τροφῇ καὶ ἀναπαύσει. ἐπὴν πίῃ ἐλλέβορον, πρὸς τὰς κινήσιας τῶν σωμάτων μᾶλλον ἄγειν, μὴ πρὸς ὕπνους. δηλοῖ δὲ ἡ ναυτιλίη ὅτι κίνησις τὰ σώματα ταράσσει. ἐπὴν βούλῃ μᾶλλον ἄγειν ἐλλέβορον, κίνει τὰ σώματα. ἐλλέβορος ἐπικίνδυνος τοῖσι σάρκας ὑγιᾶς ἔχουσι. ὅσοι ἐν τῇσι φαρμακοποσίῃσιν μὴ διψῶσι, καθαιρόμενοι οὐ παύονται πρὶν ἢ διψήσωσι. σπασμὸς ἐξ ἐλλεβόρου θανάσιμον. ἐπὶ ὑπερκαθάρσει σπασμὸς ἐπιγενόμενος κακόν. ἐν τῇσι ταραχῇσι τῆς κοιλίης καὶ τοῖσιν ἐμέτοισι τοῖσιν αὐτομάτως γινομένοισιν, ἢν μὲν οἷα δεῖ καθαίρεσθαι καθαίρωνται, ξυμφέρει τε καὶ εὐφόρως φέρουσιν· εἰ δὲ μή, τοὐναντίον. ὡς δὲ ἔφην ἐν τῷ Προγνωστικῷ, κάθαρσις εὐθετεῖ ἡ ἄνω, ἐφ' ᾧ ἀπυρέτῳ ἀσιτίη, καρδιωγμὸς ἢ σκοτόδινος ἢ στόμα ἐκπικρούμενον, καθόλου τῇσιν ὑπὲρ τῶν φρενῶν ὀδύνῃσιν. ἡ δὲ κάτω, ὅπου χωρὶς πυρετοῦ στρόφος, ὀσφύος ὀδύνη, γουνάτων βάρος, καταμήνια δυσεργοῦντα, ὀδύναι ἐν τοῖσιν ὑπὸ διάφραγμα. φυλάσσεσθαι δὲ ἐν τῇσιν φαρμακοποσίῃσιν τοὺς ἀστείους τὰ σώματα, μάλιστα δὲ τοὺς μέλανας καὶ ὑγροσάρκους καὶ τοὺς ὑποξήρους δὲ καὶ ψελλοὺς καὶ τραυλούς. ὁκόσοι δὲ τὰ φλεγμαίνοντα ἐν ἀρχῇ τῆς νούσου, ὡς ἔφην ἐν τῷ Περὶ πτισάνης, εὐθέως ἐπιχειροῦσι λύειν
390 φαρμακείῃ, τοῦ μὲν ξυν|τεταμένου καὶ φλεγμαίνοντος οὐδὲν ὠφελέουσιν, οὐδὲ γὰρ διαδιδοῖ ὠμὸν ἐὸν τὸ πάθος, τὰ δὲ ἀντέχοντα τῷ νοσήματι καὶ ὑγιεινὰ ξυντήκουσι· ἀσθενέος δὲ τοῦ σώματος γινομένου τὸ νόσημα ἐπικρατεῖ, καὶ ἀνιήτως ἔχουσι. ἐλλεβορίζειν δὲ χρὴ οἷσιν ἀπὸ κεφαλῆς φέρεται ῥεῦμα. μὴ διδόναι δὲ ἐπὶ ἐμπύων. μὴ φαρμακεύειν τοὺς ἀχρόους, τοὺς βραγχώδεας, τοὺς σπληνώδεας, τοὺς ἀφαίμους, τοὺς πνευματώδεας καὶ ξηρὰ βήσσοντας, διψώδεας, φυσώδεας, ἐντεταμένους ὑποχόνδρια καὶ πλευρὰς καὶ μετάφρενα, τοὺς ἀπονεναρκωμένους καὶ ἀμαυρὰ βλέποντας καὶ οἷσιν ἦχοι τῶν ὤτων καὶ τῆς οὐρήθρης ἀκρατεῖς μηδὲ τοὺς ἰκτερώδεας ἢ κοιλίης ἀσθενέας ἢ αἱμορρώδεας ἢ ἐν φύμασιν. ἢν δὲ φαρμακεῦσαι δοκῇ, ἐλλεβόρῳ ἀσφαλῶς ἄνω κάθαιρε, κάτω δὲ μή· κράτιστον δὲ τούτοισι

---

21. Mss. MUVHcb(ex p. 100, lin. 6) 3 πλείονι: πλέον ἢ U πίει U || 5 βούλει UM (corr. M[2]) ἄγει c || 6 ante σάρκας add. τὰς c || 8 διψώσωσι M post σπασμὸς add. ἢ λυγμὸς c || 11 καθαίρονται V εἰ: ἢν c || 12 εὐθετεῖ ἡ: cH εὐθετίη MUV ᾧν mss. corr. Li. || 13 post ἀσιτίη add. ἢ M[2] ἢ om. c (bis) σκοτώδινος UH στόματος U || 14 ἡ: εἰ U || 17 ὑποξύρους M || 20 τοῦ: τοὺς c ξυντεταμένους c φλεγμαίνοντας c || 21 διαδίδω M διαδίδωσιν U || 24 ἔμπυον MU ἐμπτύων c post φαρμ. add .δὲ Uc || 25 βραγχωδέους c || 28 καὶ[1] om. c οἷσιν: οἱ VMU τῶν νώτων M || 29 φυσήμασι U δοκέῃ H δοκεῖ M δοκέει c || 30 ἀσφαλὴς VM κάθαρε U

21. On treatment with hellebore, Hippocrates to Democritus.[1]

For those who are not easily purged upward, moisten their bodies before the draught with extra food and rest.[2] When one drinks hellebore, bring him more toward bodily movement, not sleep. Seasickness shows that movement disturbs bodies.[3] When you want the hellebore to bring up more, disturb the body.[4] Hellebore is dangerous for those with healthy flesh.[5] Those who are not thirsty when they have drunk the drug do not stop being purged until they are thirsty.[6] Convulsions caused by hellebore are a deadly sign.[7] Convulsion after excessive purging is bad.[8] In perturbations of the intestines and vomitings that are spontaneous, if they purge what they should, they are helpful and the patients bear it easily. If not, not.[9] As I said in *Prognostic*, purging upward is convenient for those without fever who have no appetite, who have heartburn, fainting, bitterness in the mouth, and generally for pains above the diaphragm.[10] Purging below is convenient for intestinal pain without fever, pain in the lower back, heaviness of the knees,[11] menstrual difficulties, pain below the diaphragm. In purgations, watch out for those whose bodies are in good condition, especially the dark and moist-fleshed, but also the dry, and those who stutter and lisp. Those who try to relieve inflammation immediately with purging at the beginning of the disease, as I said in *On Barley Gruel*, do not help the swelling and inflammation, for while the affection is raw it yields nothing, but they melt down the healthy parts that are resisting the disease. When the body is weakened the disease wins and they become incurable.[12] But one should give hellebore to those who have a flow from the head. And do not give it in empyema.[13] And do not purge those who have bad color, who are hoarse, have swollen spleens, are anemic, have lung problems and dry cough, are thirsty, flatulent, who have stretched hypochondria, ribs and upper back, who have torpor, whose vision is darkened, who have echoing in the ears, are incontinent of urine, nor to the jaundiced, those with weak intestines, or who have bloody stools, or in cases of tumorous swellings.[14] If you decide to purge, purge upwards safely with

---

[1] This treatise is a pastiche of statements on treatment with hellebore from the Corpus Hippocraticum, accurately transcribed, but with changes to make a coherent work. Some compatible material has been added from elsewhere.

[2] *Aph.* 4.13.

[3] *Aph.* 4.14

[4] *Aph.* 4.15.

[5] *Aph.* 4.16.

[6] *Aph.* 4.19.

[7] *Aph.* 5.1 (cf. *Coan Prognoses* 556).

[8] *Aph.* 5.4 (cf. *Coac.* 554).

[9] *Aph.* 1.2 (cf. 1.25, 4.3, *Epidemics* 6.5.1).

[10] This paraphrases *Aph.* 4.17-18. The citation of *Prog.* is false.

[11] *Aph.* 4.20. The following material (through "lisp") is not in the Corpus Hippocraticum, and has clearly post-Hippocratic language.

[12] Adapted from *Reg. in Acut. Append.* 3, 2.402 Li.

[13] *Reg. in Acut. Append.* 16, 2.474 Li.

[14] Adapted from *Reg. in Acut. Append.* 23, 2. 506-8 Li.

διαιτῶν. ὡς δὲ ἔφην ἐν τῷ Προρρητικῷ, μὴ φαρμακεύειν μηδὲ τοὺς ἐπανεμοῦντας μέλανα, ἀποσίτους καὶ παραφόρους, καθ' ἥβην σμικρὰ ὀδυνώδεας, ὄμμα θρασύ, κεκλιμένον ἔχοντας, ἐποιδοῦντας, σκοτώδεας, ἄχρους, μηδὲ τοὺς ἐν πυρετῷ καυματώδεας κατακεκλασμένους. ὡς δὲ ἔφην ἐν τῷ Περὶ πτισάνης, σησαμοειδὲς ἄνω καθαίρει. ἡ πόσις ἥμισυ δραχμῆς ἐν ὀξυμέλιτι τετριμμένον· ξυμμίσγεται δὲ καὶ τοῖσιν ἐλλεβόροισι τὸ τρίτον μέρος τῆς πόσιος καὶ ἧσσον πνίγει. καθαίρειν δὲ καὶ τοὺς ἐν χρονίοισι τεταρταίοισι καὶ τοὺς ἐν λιπυριώδει πυρετῷ χρονίους καὶ ὧν οὐκ
392 ἔστι δίψος μηδὲ ἀπόκρισις, τούτους | δὲ μὴ πρότερον τῶν τριῶν ἑβδομάδων, ποτὲ δὲ καὶ πλευριτικοὺς καὶ εἰλεώδεις· ὡς δὲ ἔφην ἐν τῷ Περὶ γυναικείων, καθαίρειν καὶ ἣν αἱ μῆτραι καθάρσεως δέωνται.

22. Ἱπποκράτους πρὸς τὸν υἱὸν Θεσσαλόν·

Ἱστορίης δὲ μελέτω σοι, ὦ παῖ, γεωμετρικῆς καὶ ἀριθμήσιος· οὐ γὰρ μόνον σέο καὶ τὸν βίον εὐκλεᾶ καὶ ἐπὶ πολλὰ χρήσιμον ἐς ἀνθρωπίνην μοίρην ἐπιτελέσει, ἀλλὰ καὶ τὴν ψυχὴν ὀξυτέρην τε καὶ τηλαυγεστέρην κατὰ τὸ ἐν ἰητρικῇ ὀνῆσθαι πᾶν ὅτι χρῄζει. καίτοι ἡ μὲν τῆς γεωμετρίης ἱστορίη, ἐοῦσα πολυσχήμων τε καὶ πολυειδὴς καὶ πᾶν μετ' ἀποδείξεως περαινομένη, ἔσται χρησίμη πρός τε τὰς τῶν ὀστέων θέσεις καὶ ἐξαρθρήσεις καὶ τὴν λοιπὴν τῶν μελέων τάξιν. ἐς τὴν γὰρ τούτων πολυτροπίην εὐεπιγνωστότερος ἐμβολῇ τε ἄρθρων καὶ τῇ τῶν ὀστέων τῶν συντριβομένων ἀναπρίσει τε καὶ ἐκτρυπήσει καὶ συνθέσει καὶ ἐξαιρέσει καὶ τῇ λοιπῇ θεραπείῃ χρῆσθαι, εἰδὼς ὁκοῖόν τε χωρίον ἐστὶ καὶ τὸ ἐκ τούτου ἐξαρθρεύμενον ὀστέον. ἡ δὲ τῆς ἀριθμήσιος τάξις πρός τε τὰς περιόδους καὶ ἀλόγους τῶν πυρετῶν μεταστάσιας καὶ τὰς κρίσιας τῶν νοσεόντων καὶ τὰς ἐν νούσοισιν ἀσφαλείας ἀρκέουσα ἔστω. μάλα γὰρ σεμνὸν ὑπηρεσίαν ἔχειν ἐν ἰητρικῇ τοιήνδε, ἥτις σοι τὰ μέρεα τῆς ἐπιτάσιος καὶ τῆς ἀνέσιος ἄνισα ἔοντα τὴν μοῖραν εὔγνωστα παρέχεται χωρὶς ἀμπλακίης. διὸ δὴ κάρτα ἐς δύναμιν ἀφίκνεο τῆς τοιῆσδε ἐμπειρίης. ἔρρωσο.

---

2 καθ' ἥβην: καθεύδειν Mss. corr. Li. ex *Prorrh. I* ‖ 3 ὀδυνώδεα V ‖ 4 καυματώδει U ‖ 5 ἐν τῷ om. MU καθαίρειν U ‖ 6 τετριμμένῳ Mss. -ον *Reg. in Acut.* ‖ 7-8 τοῖς ἐγχρονίοις V τοῖς ἐν χρον. M ‖ 9 μηδὲ: οὐδὲ H τούτους δὲ: τούσδε U ‖ 11 δέονται U

22. Mss. MUVbO(=cd) 14 ὦ παῖ ante μελέτω V ‖ 16 τε om. bO ‖ 17 ὀνῆσθαι: M ὀνεῖσθαι UO ὤνησθαι b ὠνῆσθαι V χρήζεις b ‖ 18 πολὺσχειμών corr. in πολὺ χειμών M πολυσχημός UO ‖ 19 ἔστω U τε om. O ‖ 19-20 καὶ ἐξαρθρήσεις om. U ἐξαριθμήσεις b[2] ‖ 20 ἐς τὴν: εἴση bO ‖ 21 ἐμβολὴ VM τῶν om. O ‖ 22 ἀναποίσει V ‖ 23 εἶδος corr. in εἰδὼς M εἰδότι U ‖ 24 ἐξαρθρεύμενον: scripsi ἐξορεύμενον MVb ἐξορώμενον U ἐξαιρεύμενον b[2] ἐξερεύμενον O τε om. O ‖ 26 τὰς: τῆς mss. corr. Li. ἔστω: ἑκάστῳ d ἔσται b[2] ‖ 27 ἐπιστάσιος M ‖ 28 τῆς om. O ἄνισα ἐόντα τὴν: ἐόντα ἄνισα ὄντα την (τῇ U) MUb ὄντα ἄνισα ἐς ἰσοτάτην O ἄνισα τὴν b μοῖρα U ‖ 29 ἀφικνέω U αφικνέοιο O

hellebore, not down; it is best to treat them with diet.[1] As I said in *Prorrhetic*, do not purge those who suffer from black vomit, lack of appetite, delirium, small pains in the pubis, with eye bold, partly closed, who have swelling, blindness, lack of color, nor those burning with fever, or prostrated by it.[2] And as I said in *On Barley Gruel*, sesamoid (the fruit of the black hellebore) purges up. The dose is half a dram crushed in oxymel. A third part of the drink is mixed with the hellebores and chokes less.[3] Purge those with chronic quartans, those with chronic malignant intermittent fevers, those without thirst or significant excretions, but not before three seven-day periods. Sometimes also those with pleurisy and iliac problems.[4] And as I said in *On Women's Diseases*, purge if the womb needs purging.[5]

22. Hippocrates to his son Thessalos. Greetings.

Devote yourself, my child, to the study of geometry and numbers. Not only will it make your life respectable and effective in many ways with respect to the human condition, but it will improve your intellect, make it more quick and far-sighted for achieving anything you want to do in medicine. The study, indeed, of geometry, being many-shaped and multiformed and proceeding wholly by demonstration, will be useful for positioning bones, articulating them, and for all other orderings of the limbs. In the variety of these matters a physician is more adept at setting the joints, sawing off shattered bones, and boring holes, putting them in place and removing them and all other therapeutic measures, if he knows the nature of the place and of the bone that has been displaced from it.

And in relation to cycles, irrational alterations of fevers, and crises of the ill, let orderly calculations assist for safety in disease. For it is a noble thing to have such assistance in medicine: it renders, unerringly, easily intelligible those portions of intensification and remission, which are unequal in their fate.

Wherefore, do enter into the power of such knowledge. Be well!

---

[1] Adapted from *Reg. in Acut. Append.* 25, 2.510 Li.

[2] Adapted from *Prorrhetic* 1.71, 5.528 Li.

[3] *Reg. in Acut. Append.* 28, 2.514-16 Li.

[4] This material is related to a discussion of *causus* in *Critical Days*, Littré 9.280.

[5] This is not a quotation from a known work, though it is suggestive of *Aph.* 5.36, *Nature of Woman* 23 (7.342 Li.), and *Diseases of Women 1*.16 (8.54 Ll.), *1*.74 (8.156-8 Li.), 2.110 (8.238 Li.).

23. Δημόκριτος Ἱπποκράτει περὶ φύσεως ἀνθρώπου

394 Χρὴ πάντας ἀνθρώπους ἰητρικὴν τέχνην ἐπίστασθαι, ὦ Ἱππόκρα|τες· καλὸν γὰρ ἅμα καὶ ξυμφέρον ἐς τὸν βίον, τούτων δὲ μάλιστα τοὺς παιδείας καὶ λόγων ἴδριας γεγενημένους. ἱστορίην σοφίης γὰρ δοκέω ἰητρικῆς ἀδελφὴν καὶ ξύνοικον. σοφίη μὲν γὰρ ψυχὴν ἀναρύεται παθέων, ἰητρικὴ δὲ νούσους σωμάτων ἀφαιρεῖται. αὔξεται δὲ νοῦσος παρεούσης ὑγείης, ἣν καλὸν προνοεῖν τοὺς ἐσθλὰ φρονέοντας· ἕξεως δὲ σωματικῆς ἀλγεούσης οὐδὲ προθυμίην ἄγει νόος ἐς μελέτην ἀρετῆς· νοῦσος γὰρ παρεοῦσα δεινῶς ψυχὴν ἀμαυροῖ, φρόνησιν ἐς συμπαθείην ἄγουσα. φύσεως δὲ ἀνθρωπίνης ἡ περιγραφὴ θεωρίην ἔχει τοιήνδε· ὁ μὲν ἐγκέφαλος φρουρεῖ τὴν ἄκρην τοῦ σώματος, ἀσφάλειαν ἐμπεπιστευμένος, ὑμέσι νευρώδεσι συνεισκατοικέων, ὑπὲρ ὧν ὀστέων διπλαῖ φύσιες ἀναγκαίῃ ἀρηρυῖαι δεσπότην, φύλακα διανοίης καλύπτουσιν, ἐγκέφαλον, τριχῶν εὐκοσμίαι χρῶτα κοσμεῦσι. τὸ δὲ τῶν ὀμμάτων ὁρητικὸν ἐν πολυχίτωνι φωλεῦον ὑγροῦ ἐνστασίᾳ ὑπὸ μέτωπον κοιλασίῃ συνίδρυται, θεωρίης δὲ αἴτιον. ἀκριβὴς δὲ κόρη φύλακα ταρσὸν εὐκαιρίης ὑπομένει. διπλοῖ δὲ ῥώθωνες, ὀσφρήσιος ἐπιγνώμονες, διορίζουσιν ὀφθαλμῶν γειτνίην. μαλακὴ δὲ χειλέων ἀφὴ στόματι περιπτυσσομένη, ῥημάτων αἴσθησιν ἀκριβῆ τε διάρθρωσιν παρέσχηκεν κυβερνωμένη. γένειον δὲ ἀκροτελὲς καὶ χελύνειον γόμφοισι συνηρμοσμένον. ἐνδοχεῖα δὲ μύθων ὦτα δημιουργὸς ἀνέῳγεν, οἷσιν ἐπεὼν ὁ θυμὸς οὐκ ἀσφαλὴς διήκονος ἀλογιστίης γίνεται. λαλιῆς μήτηρ γλῶσσα, ψυχῆς ἄγγελος, πυλωρεῦσα τὴν γεῦσιν, ἐχυροῖσιν ὀδόντων θριγκοῖσι πεφρούρηται. βρόγχος δὲ καὶ φάρυγξ ἡρμοσμένοι ἀλλήλοισι γειτνιῶσιν· ὁ μὲν γὰρ ἐς κέλευθον πνεύματος, ὁ δὲ ἐς βυθὸν
396 κοιλίης τροφὴν προπέμπει λάβρον ὠθεύμενος. κω|νοειδὴς δὲ καρδίη βασιλίς, ὀργῆς τιθηνὸς πρὸς πᾶσαν ἐπιβουλήν, ἐνδέδυκε θώρακα. θαμιναὶ δὲ πνευμάτων σήραγγες, ἠέρι διοδεύμεναι, φωνῆς αἴτιον πνεῦμα τίκτουσιν. τὸ δὲ χορηγὸν αἵματος καὶ μεταβάλλον τὴν τροφὴν σὺν λοβοῖσι πολλάκις κοιλῇ περίπλοον ἔσται ἧπαρ ἐπιθυμίης αἴτιον. χλωρὴ δὲ χολὴ πρὸς ἥπατι μένουσα καὶ διαφθορὴ σώματος ἀνθρωπηΐου ὑπερβλύσασα γίνεται. βλαβερὸς δὲ σώματος ἀνθρωπίνου καὶ ἀνωφελὴς ἔνοικος σπλὴν ἀπέναντι εὕδει πρᾶγμα μηδὲν αἰτούμενος. μέση δὲ τούτων χορηγεῖ πανδέκτειρα κοιλίη, κατευνάζεται διοικέουσα τὴν πέψιν. ἔνοχα δὲ κοιλίης, συνθέσεως δημιουργίῃ συνδεσμεύμενα, εἱλεῖται περὶ κοιλίην ἔντερα, λήψεως καὶ ἀποκρίσεως αἴτια. δίδυμοι δὲ νεφροὶ ἰσχίοισιν ἐνηδρασμένοι καὶ ἠμφιεσμένοι δημῷ οὔρων ἐκκρίσεως οὐκ ἀλλότριοι

---

23. Mss. bcH 3 ξυμφορον b^2 ‖ 10 ἡπεργραφὴ b ὑπεργραφὴ cH corr. Putz. ‖ 12 ὃν bc ἀναγκαίαι b ἀναγκαῖαι cH ‖ 13 εὐκοσμία cH ‖ 14 κοσμῶσαι bcH correxi ‖ 15 ἐνστασίαις bcH corr. Diels. κολασίῃ bcH corr. Diels. ‖ 16 ὑπομένειν bcH corr. Li. ‖ 19 περιέσχε c ἀκροτενὲς b^2 ‖ 23 τριγχοῖσι b τριχοῖοι cH corr. Com. ‖ 25 κωνοειδὲς bc ‖ 28 μετάβαλον c τὴν: εἰς c ‖ 29 κοιλὴ bH περίπλοος bcH correxi χολὴ δὲ χλωρὴ H ‖ 30-31 ἀνθρωπηΐου...σώματος om. H ‖ 33 δ' ἔνυχα δὲ bcH corr. Com. ‖ 34 συνδονεύμενα c ‖ 35 λείψεως c ‖ 36 δήμοι bc δῆμοι H corr. Foës

23. Democritus to Hippocrates. On the Nature of Man.

All men should know the science of medicine, Hippocrates (it is a beautiful thing, useful to life) especially those men engaged in education and reasoning. The search for wisdom is, I think, the sister and companion of medicine. For wisdom draws the soul back from passions and medicine takes away the body's ills. Disease develops when health is present, and it is proper for right thinking men to foresee that. But as soon as the state of the body is ill, the mind brings no eagerness to the practice of virtue. The presence of disease powerfully darkens the soul by turning the intellect towards sympathetic affection.[1]

Of man's nature the outline has this aspect. The brain guards the acropolis of the body, the trustee of its safety, housed in tendinous tissues. Over them a twofold growth of bone, fitted by necessity, conceals the ruler, guardian of the intellect, the brain. An elegance of hair decorates the skin. The visual faculty of the eyes, lurking in a many coated abode of moisture is established beneath the brow, in a hollow, and is the cause of sight. The precise pupil accepts the woven lid as guardian of her proper times. The pair of nostrils, supervisors of smell, mark off the neighborhood of the eyes. The soft touch of the lips, folded about the mouth, by its supervision offers accurate articulation and perception of speech. The projecting chin is a tortoise shell bolted on. He who made us opened our ears as receivers of tales. The passion that is in them is an undependable servant of irrationality. The tongue is the mother of talk, messenger of the soul, gatekeeper of taste. She is guarded by a firm battlement of teeth. The windpipe and gullet, adapted to each other, are nearby. One gives onto the path of the wind, the other conducts food to the depth of the belly, with a firm push. Conical, the royal heart, nurse of anger against all schemes, resides in the chest. The many caves of the winds, channels for air, produce the breath that is the cause of speech. The organ that supplies the blood, which alters the food with its lobes, will often wrap around the hollow (vein), the liver, cause of passions. The yellow bile stays by the liver and when it overflows becomes the ruination of man's body. The harmful spleen, useless inhabitant of man's body sleeps opposite, responsible for nothing. And between them their mistress, the all-receiving belly has her couch, supervising the digestion. Attached to the stomach joined in artisanry of construction, the intestines are coiled about the belly, the cause of reception and division. The twin kidneys firmly established in the loins and clothed in fat, are not foreign to excreting urine.

---

[1] The author of this letter seems to have made up this phrase, and Johannes Chrysostom seems to have been impressed by it: "Do you not hear the doctors saying 'νόσος γὰρ παροῦσα δεινῶς ψυχὴν ἀμαυροῖ;' *In acta apostolorum homiliae*, Migne 60.32.39-40. Susceptibility of the soul to the body's affections was, of course, an important philosophical as well as medical question, as is shown by Galen's *Quod animi mores corporis temperamenta sequantur*, Galen, *Scr. min.* 2, 32-79.

πεφύκασι. κύριος δὲ ἁπάσης κοιλίης ὁ καλούμενος ἐπίπλους γαστέρα πᾶσαν ἐμπεριείληφεν, μόνου σπληνὸς ἄτερ. ἑξῆς νευρώδης κύστις ἰσχίῳ στόμα ἐνηδρασμένη, συμπεπλεγμένων ἀγγείων, οὔρων ἐκκρίσεως αἰτίη γίγνεται. ἡ δὲ γειτνιῶσα ταύτῃ μήτηρ βρεφέων ἤ, δεινὸν ἄλγος, τῶν ἐν γυναικὶ μόχθων μυρίων παραιτίη, μήτρη πεφώλευκεν· ἡ πυλωρὸς μυχοῖσιν ἰσχίων βράσασα σὰρξ σφίγγεται νεύροισιν, ἐκ δὲ πλήθους ἐκχέουσα γαστρὸς φύσιος, ἐκ τόκου προνοίης. ἐκ δὲ σώματος κρεμαστοὶ ἐκτὸς οἰκίην νέμονται ἐκγονοκτίσται ὄρχεις πολυχίτωνες ἐόντες. σὺν οἷσιν ἐν ἥβῃ ἀπὸ
398 φλεβέων τε καὶ νεύρων | πλέγμα οὔρων ἔκχυσιν ποιεύμενον, συνουσίης ὑπουργόν, φύσιος ὕπο δεδημιούργηται, θριξὶν ἥβης πυκαζόμενον. σκέλη δὲ καὶ βραχίονες καὶ τὰ προσηρτημένα τούτοισιν ἄκρα, διηκονίης πᾶσαν ἀρχὴν συνηθροισμένα ἔχοντα, νεύρων τε ἀσφαλῆ λειτουργίην τελέουσιν. ἡ δὲ ἀσώματος ἐν μυχοῖσι φύσις ἐξέτευξε παντάμορφα σπλάγχνων γένη, ἃ δὴ θάνατος ἐπισταθεὶς ὠκέως ἔπαυσε λειτουργίης.

24. Ἱπποκράτους ὑγιεινὸν πρὸς Δημήτριον βασιλῆα

Ἱπποκράτης Κῷος βασιλεῖ Δημητρίῳ χαίρειν·

Ἡμεῖς καὶ πρότερον μὲν σπουδάζοντες, ὦ βασιλεῦ, περὶ τῆς ἀνθρωπίνης φύσιος ἐν κεφαλαίῳ θεωρῆσαι τὰ μέρη, ταῦτα ξυγγράψαντες, καθάπερ ἠξίωσας, ἀπεστείλαμεν. νῦν δὲ περὶ ὧν δεῖ μάλιστα σπουδάζειν τοὺς ἔμφρονας, ἡμεῖς τὰ μὲν καὶ παρὰ τῶν πρότερον παρειληφότες, τὰ δὲ καὶ νῦν αὐτοὶ προσεξευρίσκοντες γεγράφαμέν σοι. οἷσι σὺ τῶν προτέρων ἀρρωστημάτων σημείοισι γινομένοισιν ἐπακολουθῶν καὶ χρώμενος πλειστάκις ἄνουσος ἂν εἴης τὸν ἅπαντα χρόνον. ἔστι δὲ δύο γένη ἀρρωστιῶν ἁπάντων ζῴων· ἡ μὲν κατὰ γένος, ἡ δὲ κατὰ πάθος, ἀνόμοιαι. τὰς δ' ἐπιθυμίας τὰς κατὰ τὴν τροφὴν ἐκ τῶν ὑπεναντίων ὄψει ξηραινομένων ⟨τὰ μὲν ὑγρά⟩, τῶν κενουμένων τὰ δὲ πλήρη, πληρούντων δὲ κενά. τὰς δὲ νούσους ἁπάσας ἐξ ὑπεναντίων ὄψει καθεστηκυίας καὶ νούσους ὑπὸ νούσων λυομένας. ὑπὸ σπασμῶν πυρετὸς ἐπιγενόμενος ἵστησι τὸ νόσημα. κεφαλῆς πολλὰς δὲ περιωδυνίας τὰ κατὰ τὰ ὦτα ῥαγέντα ἢ κατὰ τὰς ῥῖνας. [σπασμοὶ] πᾶσι δὲ μελαγχολικοῖσιν αἱμορροΐδες ἐπιγινόμεναι παύουσι τὰς μελαγχολίας. καὶ καθόλου μέν ἐστιν καὶ ῥίζα
400 τῶν ἀνθρωπίνων νοσημάτων ἡ κεφαλή, καὶ | τὰ ἀρρωστήματα τὰ μέγιστα ἐκ ταύτης παραγίνεται. ἐπικειμένην γὰρ αὐτὴν τῷ στόματι ὥσπερ σικύαν τῶν ἐσφερομένων ἁπάντων συμβαίνει αὐτὴν ἕλκειν περιττώματα καὶ τοὺς λεπτομερεῖς χυμούς. δεῖ δὲ προσέχειν

---

7 γαστρὸς: ὑστρὸς b[2] || 8 ἔκγονοι κτίσται bcH corr. Diels. σὺν οἷσιν ἐν ἥβῃ: scripsi εὔνοι ἥβη bc εὐνοίης ἥβη H || 10 ὑποδεδημιούργηται bcH corr. Li. θριξὶν: ὄρεξιν c || 13 ἐξέταξε c || 14 ἐπιστραφὲς c

24. Mss. bc (Littré's Ms. D gets its text from Cornarius, Basel 1538) 17 μὲν om. c || 20 σώφρονας cb[2] ἠληφότες c || 23-4 δύο γένη…ἡ δὲ om. c || 26 τὰ μὲν ὑγρά: addidi om. mss. edd. || 27-8 ἐξ…πυρετὸς om. c || 28 λυομένας: Ilberg γινομένας mss. edd. || 29 πολλῆς bc -ὰς Foës in not. τὰ[1]: scripsi ὅταν bc αἷμα Corn. || 30 σπασμοὶ seclusi αἱμορροΐδες om. c || 31 ἐπιγινόμεναι: scripsi -οι mss., edd. καὶ[1] om. c || 32 ἡ om. c || 33 σώματι Corn. || 34 σικύ b corr. b[2]

Presiding over the whole belly the peritoneum, as it is called, surrounds the whole belly save the spleen alone. Next is the sinewy bladder established with its mouth in the groin, of woven vessels, the cause of excretion of urine. As neighbor to it, lurks the mother of babes, who, dread pain, is contributor of myriad difficulties in women, the womb. Her gate, seething flesh in the hollows of the groin, is wrapped in sinew, and it pours forth from excess of the belly's nature, in her anticipation of children. And hanging away from the body, the testicles, fashioners of offspring, make their home on the outside; they have many coats. With them on the pubis, a woven construction of veins and sinews, which accomplishes the outpour of urine and is the assistant in sex, was crafted by nature, surrounded by a thicket of pubic hair. The legs and arms and the tips attached to them collectively have all the source of ministry, and perform unerringly the service assigned by the nerves. But it is the incorporeal nature in the inner parts who fashions multiformed types of organs. Death, when it comes nigh, swiftly ends their service.

24. Hippocrates' *Hygiene* for King Demetrius.

Hippocrates of Cos to King Demetrius. Greetings.[1]

Earlier having been concerned to arrive at a summary view of the parts of the human organism, I composed it and sent it to you at your request, king. Now, concerning what intelligent men must especially be concerned with, having taken some things from my predecessors and having myself made additional discoveries I have written it for you. Following and using this and the signs from previous illnesses, you will always be generally free from sickness.

Illnesses in all living creatures are of two varieties, one disease is according to type, the other according to the affection, and they are dissimilar, You will see that desires for nutriment spring from opposites, the dry desiring the wet, the empty the full, the full the empty. And you will see that all diseases arise from opposites, and that diseases resolve diseases. Fever supervening from convulsions puts down the disease,[2] and flows breaking forth from nose or ears put an end to severe head pain.[3] And in all melancholics hemorrhoids coming on stop melancholy.[4] And generally the head is the root of human ills, and the greatest sicknesses come from it. For, placed over the mouth like a cupping glass,[5] it is its fate to draw the excrement and the thin humors from all ingested material.

Having accustomed yourself to live in a private way, you must pay attention to

---

[1] This is the least literate of the letters, and it has the weakest manuscript evidence: one of the three manuscripts (D = Par. Graec. 2444) is in this treatise a copy of Cornarius' printed text of 1538. Its existence in ms. b, however, insures that it is not a production of the Renaissance.

[2] Drawn from *Aph.* 4.57, or *Crises* 61 (Li. 9..294).

[3] Drawn from *Crises* 57 (Li. 9.292).

[4] Drawn from *Aph.* 6.11.

[5] The comparison of the head to a cupping glass is from *Diseases 4*, Li. 7.548.

τὸν νοῦν, ἰδίως ζῆν αὐτὸν παρασκευάσαντα, ἐς ταῦτα τὰ μέρη, ὅκως μηδεμίαν αὔξησιν λαμβάνοντα τὰ προσπίπτοντα τῶν ἀρρωστημάτων, διά τε τῆς ἐπιμελείης καὶ τῆς εὐταξίης τῆς παρὰ σοὶ γινομένης, καὶ μήτε τῇσι τῶν ἀφροδισίων ἀκρασίῃσι μήτε τῇσι τῶν διαφόρων ἐδεσμάτων μήτε τοῖσιν ὕπνοισι τοῖσιν ὑπερχαλαστικοῖσιν ἀγυμνάστου ἔοντος τοῦ σώματος χρώμενον, ἀλλ' ἐπακολουθοῦντα τοῖσι σημείοισι τοῖσι γιγνομένοισιν ἐν τῷ σώματι διατηρεῖν τὸν καιρὸν ἕκαστον σώματος, ὅκως ἂν φυλαξάμενος τὸ ἀρρώστημα τὸ μέλλον ἐπιφέρεσθαι, τῇσι θεραπείῃσιν ᾗσιν ἂν ἐγὼ γράφω χρώμενος διατελῇς ἄνουσος ἐών.

25. Δόγμα Ἀθηναίων.

Ἔδοξε τῇ βουλῇ καὶ τῷ δήμῳ τῶν Ἀθηναίων. ἐπειδὴ Ἱπποκράτης Κῷος, ἰατρὸς ὑπάρχων καὶ γεγονὼς ἀπὸ Ἀσκληπιοῦ, μεγάλην εὔνοιαν μετὰ σωτηρίας ἐνδέδεικται τοῖς Ἕλλησιν, ὅτι καὶ λοιμοῦ ἰόντος ἀπὸ τῆς βαρβάρων ἐπὶ τὴν Ἑλλάδα, κατά τε τόπους ἀποστείλας τοὺς αὐτοῦ μαθητὰς παρήγγειλε τίσι χρὴ θεραπείαις χρωμένους ἀσφαλῶς διασώσεσθαι τὸν ἐπιόντα λοιμόν, ὅπως τε ἰατρικὴ δοθεῖσα τοῖς Ἕλλησιν ἀσφαλῶς σῴζῃ τοὺς κάμνοντας αὐτόν, ἐξέδωκε δὲ καὶ ξυγγραφὰς ἀφθόνως τὰς περὶ τῆς ἰατρικῆς τέχνης, πολλοὺς βουλόμενος τοὺς σῴζοντας ὑπάρχειν ἰατρούς· τοῦ τε Περσῶν βασιλέως μεταπεμπομένου αὐτὸν ἐπὶ
402 τιμαῖς ταῖς κατ' αὐτὸν | ἴσαις καὶ δώροις ἐφ' οἷς ἂν αὐτὸς Ἱπποκράτης αἱρῆται, ὑπερεῖδε τὰς ὑποσχέσεις τοῦ βαρβάρου, ὅτι πολέμιος καὶ κοινὸς ἐχθρὸς ὑπῆρχε τοῖς Ἕλλησιν. ὅπως οὖν ὁ δῆμος Ἀθηναίων φαίνηται προαιρούμενος τὰ χρήσιμα διὰ παντὸς ὑπὲρ τῶν Ἑλλήνων καὶ ἵνα χάριν ἀποδῷ πρέπουσαν Ἱπποκράτει ὑπὲρ τῶν εὐεργετημάτων, δέδοκται τῷ δήμῳ μυῆσαι αὐτὸν τὰ μυστήρια τὰ μεγάλα δημοσίᾳ καθάπερ Ἡρακλέα τὸν Διός, καὶ στεφανῶσαι αὐτὸν στεφάνῳ χρυσῷ ἀπὸ χρυσῶν χιλίων· ἀναγορεῦσαί τε τὸν στέφανον Παναθηναίοις τοῖς μεγάλοις ἐν τῷ ἀγῶνι τῷ γυμνικῷ· καὶ ἐξεῖναι πᾶσι Κώων παισὶν ἐφηβεύειν ἐν Ἀθήναις ἐπειδήπερ ἡ πατρὶς αὐτῶν ἄνδρα τοιοῦτον ἐγέννησεν· εἶναι δὲ Ἱπποκράτει καὶ πολιτείαν καὶ σίτησιν ἐν Πρυτανείῳ διὰ βίου.

---

5 ὑπερκολαστικοῖς bc ὑπερκαλυστικοῖς b^2 corr. Li. post ὑπερκ. add. καὶ c ‖ 6 χρώμενος bc corr. Li. ‖ 9 διατελεῖς bc corr. Foës ‖ 7 ἕκαστον: A.J. Graham ἑκάστου mss. edd.

25. Mss. MUVbc 12 ἰητρὸς bc ‖ 13 ὅτι: scripsi ὅτε MUVbc ὅστις b^2 καὶ om. U ‖ 14 τε om. MVbc ‖ 15 παρήγγειλε: παρήγγελλεν b om. V τῇσι V χρὴ θεραπείαις MUV δεῖ (δὲ c) χρῆσθαι θεραπείαις αἷς bc ‖ 16 διασώσεσθαι: διασώζεσθαι b(corr. b^2)c διαφεύξευσθαι U post ἰητρικὴ add. τέχνη U τέχνη ἀπόλλωνος (ἀπόλλω b) bc διαδοθεῖσα Ubc ‖ 17 σώζει U αὐτῶν MUb συγγράψαι c ξυγγράψας MVb συγγραφὰς U ‖ 18 ἀφθόνως: ἀφειδῶς Mbc ἀκριβῶς U τάς: τὰ MVbc ἰατρικῆς: MU ἰητρικῆς Vbc ‖ 19 ἰητροὺς ὑπάρχειν U περσέων b ‖ 21 αἱρεῖται c ante πολέμιος add. καὶ bc ‖ 22 post δῆμος add. ὁ bc ‖ 24 περὶ bc δεδόκηται M^2 δεδόχθω b ‖ 25 δάμω M (corr. M^2) τὰ μεγάλα μυστήρια bc δημοσίων b δημό V ‖ 26 χρυσέω b ‖ 27 ἀναγορεύσετε M (-αιτε M^2) ἀναγορεῦσαι δὲ bc ‖ 28 παρ' ἀθηναίοις U post Ἀθήναις add. καθάπερ παισὶν (corr. ex πασὶν) Ἀθηναίων bc ‖ 30 διὰ τέλους cb (corr. b^2)

those parts, so that diseases that do befall you receive no increase because of your care and excellent regulation, and your abstaining from sexual excesses, excesses in variety of foods, and excesses of very relaxing sleep while your body is without exercise. Rather, following the signs that appear in the body, study each of the body's crucial moments so that, having taken preventive measures against the disease that is going to be brought on, using the remedies I describe, you will live free from disease.

25. Decree of the Athenians. The Council and the People of Athens have decreed:

Whereas Hippocrates of Cos, being a physician and descended from Asclepius, has shown great concern for the safety of the Greek people,

And whereas on the occasion of a plague coming from the land of the barbarians towards Hellas, he sent out his pupils to different places to proclaim what therapies they had to use to keep themselves safe from the imminent plague, and, in order that medical science bequeathed to the Greeks would preserve safe those that were ill from it he generously published his writings on medical science because he wanted there to be many physicians who saved people,

And when the Persian King sent for him on condition of honors equal to his own, and on condition of whatever gifts Hippocrates chose, he scorned the promises of the barbarian because he was a foe and the common enemy of Greeks,

Therefore, so that the Athenian people may show itself to desire the best always for the Greeks and so that they may show proper gratitude to Hippocrates for his beneficent acts,

It is decreed by the people to initiate him into the great mysteries at public expense as was done with Heracles, the son of Zeus,

And to crown him with a gold crown worth one thousand gold pieces, and to proclaim the crown at the great Panathenaia at the athletic competition,

And that it be permitted to all sons of the Coans to be ephebes in Athens, since their country has begotten such a man,

And that there be for Hippocrates citizenship, and sustenance in the Prytaneum for his lifetime.

26. Ἐπιβώμιος

Ὦ πολλοὶ καὶ πολλῶν πολίων οἰκηταί, ἐν ἀξίῃ μεγάλῃ γεγῶτες, κοινὸν οὔνομα Θεσσαλοί, πᾶσιν ἀνθρώποισι πικρὴ ἀνάγκη τὰ μεμοιραμένα φέρειν· καρτερεῖν γὰρ βιάζεται ἃ βούλεται. εἰ καὶ νῦν ἐγὼ εἴκων, ξὺν ἐμῇ γενεῇ θαλλοὺς στέψας, ἐπ' Ἀθηναίης βωμοῦ ἱκέτης ἵδρυμαι, τίς ἐὼν χρὴ λέγειν τοῖσιν ἀγνοέουσιν. Ἱπποκράτης, ὦ ἄνδρες, ὁ ἰητρός. ὁμοίως οὐ διὰ σεμνῆς καὶ καλῆς αἰτίης ἐμὲ ἐμεωυτὸν καὶ παῖδας ὑμῖν ξυνίστημι. γινώσκεσθε, ὦ πληθύς· καὶ γὰρ δή, ὦ ἄνδρες οἰκεῖοι, ἐν οἷσιν, ὡς εἰπεῖν
404 ἀληθές, πολλοῖσιν ὑμέων | καὶ πολίων ὑμετέρων γινώσκομαι. ὡς τύπῳ εἰπεῖν, οὔνομα δ' ἰδέης καὶ προσωτέρω κεχώρηκε, δοκέω δὲ τοῦτο ἐκ τέχνης ἐμῆς ὑγιείης τε καὶ ζωῆς αἴτιον ἀνθρώποισιν· οὐ μόνον τοῖσι τὴν ὑμετέρην οἰκέουσιν, ἀλλὰ καὶ πολλοῖσιν Ἑλλήνων ἐγγὺς ὑμέων γινώσκομαι. ἤδη διότι ἐγὼ ὑπέμεινα τὸ τηλικοῦτον πρῆγμα ἔργῳ πρᾶξαι, ἐρέω. Ἀθηναῖοι, ὦ ἄνδρες Θεσσαλοί, κακῶς ἐξουσίῃ χρεώμενοι, μητρόπολιν ἡμετέρην Κῶ ἐν δούλης μέρει διατίθενται, τὰ ἐλεύθερα διὰ προγόνων κτήσιος ἰδιόκτητα ποιεύμενοι, οὔτε ξυγγενείην αἰδεσθέντες, ἥ ἐστιν αὐτοῖσιν ἀπὸ Ἀπόλλωνός τε καὶ Ῥοιοῦς, ἥτις ἐς Ἄνιόν τε καὶ Σούνιον τοὺς κείνων παῖδας ἱκνεῖται, οὔθ' Ἡρακλέους εὐεργεσιῶν εἵνεκεν πραΰνσεας ἐς νόον βαλόμενοι ἃς ὁ κοινὸς ὑμῖν τε καὶ ἡμῖν ὀρθῶς ποιέων θεὸς ἐς ἐκείνους κατέθετο. ὑμεῖς τε ἀλλὰ πρὸς Διὸς ἱκεσίου καὶ θεῶν ὁμογνίων ἐξέλθετε, ἀμύνατε, ἐλευθερώσατε, τῆς ἰδίης φιλοτιμίης μηδὲν ἐλλείποντες.

---

26. Mss. AMUV 2 πόλεων MUV(corr M^2) οἰκηταί om. A γεγονότες AM ‖ 3 μικρὴ A μεμοιρημένα MV(corr. M^2) ‖ 4 καρτερεῖ MUV βιάζεσθαι mss. corr. Li ἅ: εἰ A. βούληται M εἰκὼν V ἥκων U ἧκον A^2 ‖ 5 ἐμοὶ γενεὰ U Ἀθηνοίοις U βώμους A ἱκέτις A ‖ 6 ἀγνωέουσιν M ὅμοι ὡς οὐ A ὁ Κῷος Cornarius ‖ 8 γινώσκεσθε scripsi -θαι mss. ὡς πληθοῦς A ὦ πλῆθος U ‖ 9 ἀληθῶς V ‖ 10 δ' εἰδέης M δὲ ἰδέης A δοκέει M δοκεῖ U ‖ 12 ἡμετέρην UA^2 post οἰκέουσιν add. ἀλλὰ καὶ πολλὴν A ‖ 13 διότι ἐγὼ scripsi δὲ ὀτέω A δὲ ὅτι ἐγω MUV ὑπεμεινάτε A ‖ 13-14 πρᾶξαι ἐρέω om. A ‖ 14 ὦ: om. A ἐξουσίῃ: Li. ἔχουσιν A ἔξουσιν M ἔξουσι U ἔχουσιν ἢ V ‖ 15 μερίδι τίθενται V μέρει διατίθεται AM(corr. M^2) μέρει διατίθεσθαι U ‖ 16 ἰδιόκτητα: δορίκτεα V (ἴδια δορίκτητα Putz.) ‖ 17 Ῥοιοῦς A Ἡρακλέους MUV Αἰνίον mss. Ἄνιόν Paton ‖ 18 κείνων: κινῶν M ἱκνέεσθαι A ‖ 19 περιῆος νόον A περιηος νόον M περι ἐς νόον V περὶ ἰὸν νοον U locus corruptus πραΰνσεας scripsi ex. gr. ‖ 20 τε: δὲ A post Διός add. τε V εἰκεσίου A ‖ 21 ἐξέλθατε AM ‖ 22 μηδὲ U ἐλλίποντες M ἐνάπτοντες A ἐλλοίτοντες U

26. Speech at the Altar.

You many inhabitants of many towns, men of great merit who bear the common name Thessalians, bitter to all men is the necessity of bearing what fate has decreed, for it forces us to acquiesce in what it wants. If I yield now to that necessity, and, along with my family take up suppliant boughs and declare myself a suppliant at Athena's altar, it is needful to tell those who do not know, who I am.

I am Hippocrates the physician. Likewise I tell you that it is not for a pompous or specious petition that I put myself and my children before you. Know that, oh people. For, my friends, among whom I can truly say I am known to many of you and many of your cities, and to speak figuratively, my name has traveled even more widely than my form, and that, I think, is because out of my science comes the cause of health and life for men: not only to those in your country but to those many Greeks in your vicinity am I known.

Now, I shall tell you why, in fact, I have submitted to doing such an extraordinary thing. The Athenians, oh men of Thessaly, using their power wrongly, have put our mother city Cos in the portion of a slave. What was free through the possessions of our ancestors they have made their private possession, showing no reverence for the kinship that they have from Apollo and Rhoio, which came down to Anius and Sunius their sons. Nor do they bring to mind, for the sake of Heracles' generosity, gentleness which the god who is common to you and to us rightly brought into being and established for them.

Still, I beg you, will you, by the god of suppliance, Zeus, and the gods of his family, come to our aid? Help us. Free us. Do not fall short of your own sense of honor.

27. Πρεσβευτικὸς Θεσσαλοῦ Ἱπποκράτους υἱοῦ.

Προσήκειν ἡγέομαι, ὦ ἄνδρες Ἀθηναῖοι, καθιστάμενον ἐς ὑμέας καὶ μὴ γινωσκόμενον παντὶ τῷ πλήθει, πρῶτον δηλῶσαι μὲν ὅστις καὶ ὅθεν ἐστί, μετὰ δὲ ταῦτα τῶν ἄλλων λόγων ἅπτεσθαι. ἐμοὶ μὲν πατὴρ Ἱπποκράτης, ὃν ὑμεῖς γινώσκετε ἐν ἰητρικῇ ἡλίκην δύναμιν ἔχει. οὔνομα δὲ Θεσσαλός· γινώσκομαι δὲ κἀγὼ οὐκ ἐν δευτέροισιν ὑμέων, οὐδὲ
406 ὀλίγοισι, πατρὶς δέ μοι Κῶς, ἣν ὅκως ὑμῖν | οἰκείη ἐστιν ἐξ ἀρχαίων, ἕτεροι ἐροῦσιν οἵτινες ἱστορίην ἐξηγήσασθαι δυνατώτεροι. ἦλθον δὲ πεμφθεὶς ὑπὸ τοῦ πατρός, τέσσαρας ἔχων εὐεργεσίας εἰπεῖν παρ' ἡμέων ἐς ὑμέας γεγενημένας· τὴν μέν τινα παλαιὰν ἐπὶ τῶν προγόνων, κοινὴν ἐς ἅπαντας τοὺς Ἀμφικτύονας, ὧν ὑμεῖς οὐκ ἐλαχίστη μοῖρα· τὴν δ' ἑτέρην ἔτι μέζω ταύτης καὶ διικνουμένην ἐς Ἑλλήνων τοὺς πλείστους· καὶ αὗται μὲν φανήσονται τῆς πόλιος καὶ τῶν προγόνων τῶν ἐμῶν ἐοῦσαι· ἡ δὲ τρίτη τοῦ πατρὸς ἰδίη, καὶ τηλικαύτη ὅσην εἷς ἀνὴρ οὐδεὶς ὑμῖν τε καὶ πολλοῖσιν Ἑλλήνων κατέθετο· ἡ δ' ὑστάτη τῶν τεσσάρων κοινὴ τοῦ πατρὸς καὶ ἐμή, καὶ οὐκ ἔτι ἐς πλείονας, ἀλλ' ἐς ὑμᾶς αὐτοὺς διικνεομένη, ἣ πρὸς μὲν τὰς ἑτέρας εὐεργεσίας καὶ προτέρας σμικρὴ ἂν φανείη, πρὸς δὲ ἑτέρων χάριτας μετρεομένη μεγάλη. αἱ μὲν δὴ εὐεργεσίαι τοιαῦται οὕτως ἔχουσιν ἃς ἔφην εἶναι, ὡς συνελόντι εἰπεῖν, δεῖ δὲ μὴ μοῦνον φάναι, ἀλλὰ καὶ ἀποδεῖξαι ὥς εἰσιν ἀληθεῖς.

2. Ἀρχὴν οὖν τῷ λόγῳ τὴν ἀρχὴν τῶν ὑπουργιῶν ποιήσομαι, τὰ δὲ ἀρχαιότατα πρῶτα λέξω, ἐν οἷσι τάχ' ἄν με καταλάβοι μακρότερα καὶ μυθωδέστερα εἰπεῖν· ποθεῖ δέ πως ἀρχαίως λέγεσθαι. ἦν γὰρ χρόνος ὅτ' ἦν Κρίσαιον ἔθνος. ἐῴκεον μὲν περὶ τὸ Πυθικὸν ἱερόν, γῆν δ' εἶχον ἥ γε νῦν τῷ Ἀπόλλωνι καθιέρωται· καλεῖται δὲ τὸ μὲν Κρίσαιον πεδίον ᾧ Λοκροὶ παροικέουσι καὶ ᾧ Μέλαινα πρόσεισι, τὸ δὲ Κίρφιον ὄρος, ᾧ Φωκεῖς παράκεινται. οὗτοι δὲ οἱ Κρίσαιοι, γενόμενοί κοτε πολλοὶ καὶ ἰσχυροὶ καὶ πλούσιοι, τούτοισι τοῖσιν ἀγαθοῖσιν ἐπὶ κακὰ ἐχρήσαντο· ἐξυβρίσαντες γὰρ πολλὰ δεινὰ καὶ παράνομα εἰργάσαντο, ἐς τὸν θεὸν ἀσεβοῦντες, Δελφοὺς καταδουλούμενοι, προσοίκους ληζόμενοι, θεωροὺς συλέοντες,
408 γυναῖκάς τε καὶ παῖδας ἀγινέοντες, | καὶ ἐς τὰ σώματα ἐξυβρίζοντες. ἀνθ' ὧν Ἀμφικτύονες ὀργισθέντες, στράτευμα ἐς τὴν γῆν ἐμβαλόντες αὐτῶν, καὶ μάχῃ νικήσαντες, τὴν χώρην ἐδῄουν καὶ τὰς πόλιας ἐπόρθεον. ἔνθα πολλὰ καὶ ἀνόσια ποιήσαντες σχετλίων ἀπήντησαν, καὶ οὐ μείω ὧν ἔπραξαν τίνοντες· μακαριστοὶ δ' ἦσαν αὐτῶν οἱ ἐν χερσὶ τελευτήσαντες,

---

27. Mss. M(vel GHI)UV 4 post ταῦτα add. οὕτω V || 5 ἔχην U || 8 δυνατώτατοι V || 9 παρ' ὑμῶν εἰς ἡμᾶς U || 11 ἀμφικτυῶνας V || 12 Ἑλλήνων: ἀλλήλων mss. corr. Corn. || 17 τὰς προτέρας εὐεργεσίας MU || 20 ἀποδείξεως εἶναι ἀληθέες M ἀποδειξε ὡς εἶναι ἀληθοῦς U ἀποδεῖξαι ὡς εἶναι ἀλήθεες V corr. Asul. ex ms. G || 23 πᾶς ἀρχαῖος MU || 23-4 ὅτ' ἦν: ὅτι ἦν U ὅτι ἣν M || 26 προσισι M || 27 παρακέονται V κοτε: ὅτε M(corr. M[2]) τότε HI || 28 ἐπὶ: ἐπεὶ V || 29 post παράνομα add. πράγματα U || 30 πρὸς οἴκους M πληϊζόμενοι MU πληζόμενοι V corr. Asul. ex ms. G || 31 τε: δὲ MV ἄγειν ἐόντες M ἄγεν ἐῶντες U ἀγεινέοντες V || 32 post στράτευμα add. καὶ MV || 33 τὴν χώρην om. U || 34 σχετλίοις U || 34-5 μειόνων ποιήσας ὧν ἔπραξαν MV

27. The Ambassadorial Speech of Thessalos, son of Hippocrates.

I think it is fitting, Athenians, that a man who comes before you not known to the whole assembly reveal who he is and whence, before he engages in the rest of his speech. My father is Hippocrates. What ability in medicine he has, you know. My name is Thessalos. Those of you who know me are not few or insignificant. My homeland is Cos. How it has been closely related to you from ancient times others will tell you who are better able than I to relate history. I have come because my father sent me with four benefits to describe to you that we have given you. The first ancient, in the time of our ancestors, common to all the Amphictyons, of whom you were not the smallest part. The second, greater still, which came to the majority of Greeks. It will be clear that these two are benefits from my ancestors and my city. The third is from my father alone, and is such as no single man ever gave to you and to numerous Greeks. The last of the four is shared by my father and me and it came not to many Greeks, but to you yourselves. It might seem small in comparison to the previous ones, but great when measured against the kindnesses of other people. These benefits are such as I have said in a summary way. But it is not only necessary to state them but to show how they are true.

2. I shall make the beginning of my speech the beginning of the benefactions, and shall speak of the most ancient first. In this I may be constrained to speak somewhat lengthily and mythologically, but the subject wants to be told in an archaic manner. There was a time when there was a Crisean race which lived around the Pythian shrine and held land now dedicated to Apollo. The area by which the Locrians live is called the Crisean Plain. The city Melaina is there, and Mount Cirphius, by which the Phocians dwell. Once on a time, the Criseans, becoming numerous, strong, and wealthy, used their good fortune for evil purposes. They grew arrogant and performed many dreadful, illegal actions, expressing impiety towards the god, enslaving Delphi, plundering its neighbors, robbing visitors to the temple, carrying off people's wives and children, and violating their persons. The Amphictyons,[1] in anger at that, invaded their territory, and, having beaten them in battle, devastated the land and sacked their cities. In this transaction, having done many unholy deeds, they met with miserable results, and paid certainly no less than they had done. The luckiest of them were

[1] Amphictyons (also spelled Amphictions), from ἀμφικτίονες, "dwellers about", means members of a religious organization of states to service and protect shrines, etc. The best known was the Delphic, associated with the temple at Delphi, an organization of twelve states initially, which after the fifth century included all Greek states. The substance of the oath which was taken by its member states may have influenced the substance of this narrative. They swore "not to destroy any polis of the Amphictyones, or starve it out, or cut off its running water, either in war or in peace; if anyone transgresses these rules, to take the field against him and call up the Poleis, and if anyone plunders the property of the god or is privy to such robbery or has any designs against the sanctuary, to take vengeance for it with hand and foot and voice and all one's power." (From Victor Ehrenberg, *The Greek State*² (London: 1969) 120. The First Sacred War, here described, took place ca. 590 B.C.

δεύτεροι δὲ οἱ δορυάλωτοι γενόμενοι, οἳ δὲ ἐς ἑτέρην χώρην καὶ πόλιας ἐπεραιώθησαν· τὰ γὰρ σφέτερα κακὰ οὐκ εἶχον ἐν ὀφθαλμοῖσιν· οἱ δὲ αὐτοῦ μείναντες τῶν αἰχμαλώτων ἀτυχέστατοι ἦσαν, ὅσοι ᾐκίζοντο ἐν χώρῃ τῇ ἑωυτῶν ξὺν γυναιξὶ καὶ τέκνοισιν, ἀγρούς τε καὶ ἄστεα πυρὶ παραδιδόμενα ἐθεώρεον· ἔτι δὲ τούτων κάκιον διῆγον οἱ ἐν τοῖσι τείχεσι διαρκέοντες, ὁκότε τῶν εἰρημένων κακῶν ἃ μὲν ἐνέβλεπον, ἃ δ' ἐπυνθάνοντο, πλέον ἀκούοντες τῶν ἀληθέων· οὕτως γάρ που ἔθος γίνεσθαι· καὶ δὴ κακὰς ἐλπίδας σωτηρίης εἶχον.

3. Ἦν δέ σφι πόλις ἐγγὺς τούτου τοῦ τόπου μεγίστη, ὅκου νῦν ὁ ἱππικὸς ἀγὼν τίθεται, ἧς τὰ τείχη ἐπεσκευάζοντο, καὶ τοὺς ἐκ τῶν ἄλλων πόλιων διαφεύγοντας ἐδέχοντο. τὰ δὲ ἀχρεῖα ἐξέβαλον καὶ τὰ ἀναγκαῖα ἐσεκομίζοντο, καὶ διενοοῦντο ὑπομένειν, ἐλπίσαντες μήτε ἐχθρῶν μάχῃ τὴν πόλιν αἱρεθῆναι μήτε κατὰ μῆκος χρόνου. οἱ δ' Ἀμφικτύονες τὰ ἄλλα τε καθεῖλον ἐπὶ ταύτῃ τῇ πόλει φρούριον ποιησάμενοι, καὶ ἐς πολιορκίην σκευάσαντες τὸ ἄλλο στράτευμα κατὰ πόλιας ἀφῆκαν. προϊόντος δὲ τοῦ χρόνου καὶ λοιμοῦ ἐς τὸ στρατόπεδον ἐμπεσόντος καὶ τῶν στρατιωτῶν νοσεόντων, τινῶν δὲ καὶ ἀποθνησκόντων, τῶν δὲ καὶ ἐκλιπόντων τὸ φρούριον διὰ τὴν νοῦσον, οἱ Ἀμφικτύονες ἐταράσσοντο, καὶ ἄλλοι ἄλλα ἐβουλεύοντο· φιλεῖ δὲ τὰ κοινὰ οὕτω πως γίνεσθαι· τέλος δὲ ἀγανακτέοντες τῷ πάθει καὶ αὐτοὺς
410 γνωσιμαχήσαντες, τῷ θεῷ ἐπέτρεψαν καὶ ἤροντο | ὅτι χρὴ ποιεῖν. ὁ δ' ἐκέλευσε πολεμεῖν, καὶ ὑπισχνεῖτο κρατήσειν, ἢν ἐς Κῶ ἐλθόντες ἐλάφου παῖδα ἐς ἐπικουρίην ἀγάγωνται ξὺν χρυσῷ, σπεύσαντες ὡς μὴ πρότερον οἱ Κρισαῖοι ἐν τῷ ἀδύτῳ τὸν τρίποδα συλήσωσιν· εἰ δὲ μή, τὴν πόλιν οὐχ ἁλώσεσθαι. οἱ δὲ ταῦτα ἀκούσαντες καὶ ἐλθόντες ἐς Κῶ, τὰ μαντευθέντα ἀπήγγειλαν· ἀπορεύντων δὲ τῶν Κώων καὶ ἀγνοεύντων τὸ μάντευμα, ἀνέστη ἀνήρ, γένος μὲν Ἀσκληπιάδης, πρόγονος δὲ ἡμέτερος, ἰητρὸς δὲ Ἑλλήνων κράτιστος ὁμολογούμενος τῶν τότε, ὄνομά οἱ ἦν Νεβρός, ὅστις ὀνομαστὶ ἔφη τὸ θέσφατον ἥκειν πρὸς ἑωυτόν· Εἴπερ ὁ θεὸς οὕτω παρήνεσεν ὑμῖν, ἐλθόντας ἐς Κῶ ἐλάφου παῖδα ἐς ἐπικουρίην ἀγαγεῖν· Κῶς μὲν γὰρ αὕτη, τὰ δὲ ἐλάφων ἔκγονα νεβροὶ καλέονται, Νεβρὸς δέ μοι οὔνομα, ἐπικουρίη δ' ἂν ἄλλη τίς προτέρη γένοιτο στρατοπέδῳ νοσέοντι ἰητροῦ; καὶ μὴν τό τε εὐθὺ ἐχόμενον, οὐ δοκέω ὅτι τοὺς τοσοῦτον Ἑλλήνων ὑπερέχοντας ὄλβῳ ἐς Κῶ προελθόντας ἔταξεν ὁ θεὸς νόμισμα χρυσοῦν αἰτεῖν· ἀλλὰ τοῦτο τὸ θέσφατον ἐς τὴν ἐμὴν οἰκίην ἔρχεται· Χρύσος γάρ μοι κεκλέαται ἀρρένων παίδων ὁ νεώτατος· ἔστι δὲ πάντα καὶ ἰδέῃ καὶ ἐς ψυχὴν ἀρετῇ, ὡς πατέρα λέγειν, διάκριτος πολιητέων. ἐγὼ μὲν οὖν, εἰ μὴ ὑμῖν ἄλλο δοκεῖ, αὐτός τε εἶμι καὶ τὸν παῖδα ἄξω, πεντηκόντορον

---

2 ἐπεραιώθησαν: ἐβεβαιώθησαν V ‖ 3 οἰκίζοντο V ‖ 4 ἄστε M ‖ 6 ἔβλεπον MU ‖ 10 ἧς: εἰς MU ‖ 13 ἐχθρῶν: Li. ex ms. J ἐφ' ὧν MUV ‖ 16 ἀφῆκεν U ‖ 19ἐταράσσοντο: deficit ms. M, memorabo mss. HI ‖ 23 ἀγάγονται mss. corr. Com. ‖ 26 ἀποροοῦντες U ‖ 27 ἀπομάντευμα UHI δὲ om. U ‖ 29 ὀνομάζειν UV^{2}HI νομίζειν V ‖ 30 ἐλθόντες U ἐς^{II} om. V ‖ 36 πάντα καὶ εἰδέῃ VHI πάντι καὶ ἰδέῃ U ‖ 37 πολιτῶν U

those who died in combat, and, secondly, those who became the spoil of war and were carried away to another land and other cities, for they did not have their evils before their eyes. But those captives who stayed there were the most unfortunate: they were outraged in their own land with their wives and children, and watched their fields and cities given over to fire. Still worse than that was experienced by those who were holding out within the fortifications.[1] They saw some of the evils I have described and learned of the rest, and what they heard was worse than the truth, for that is how it usually is. And they had little hope of being saved.

3. But there was near to them a city of that place, a very large one, where now the equestrian contest is set. They built up its walls, and they received the fugitives from the rest of the cities. They cast out what was useless and collected inside what was needed. And they determined to endure, in the hope that the city would be taken neither by enemy action nor by length of time. But the Amphictyons razed the rest, set up a fort against the city, and sending the rest of the army back to its cities, made preparations for a siege. As time went forward and plague fell on the army and the soldiers sickened, and some died, and some left the besieging force because of sickness, the Amphictyons were troubled. Some advised one thing, others another. And so it tends to go with joint projects. But finally, rankling at their suffering and disagreeing among themselves, they turned to the god and asked what they ought to do. He bade them fight, and promised that they would win if they went to Cos and brought back for assistance a deer's child with gold, hurrying so that the Criseans did not loot the tripod in the inner sanctum beforehand. If they did not do it, the city would not be captured. When they heard that, they went to Cos and made an announcement of what the oracle had said. The Coans were at a loss and did not understand the oracle, but a man stood up, an Asclepiad by family and an ancestor of mine, by common agreement the best physician of the Greeks of that time, whose name was Fawn (Nebros). He said that he believed that the oracle was directed to him. "If in fact the god so advised you to come to Cos and fetch a deer's child for assistance, this is Cos, the offspring of deer are called fawns, and Fawn is my name. What better assistance to a sick army could there be than a physician? And as for what was joined with that, indeed, I do not believe that the god directed those who excel the Greeks so much in wealth to come to Cos to ask for gold currency. Rather this oracle comes on my house. Gold (Chrysos) is the name of my youngest male child. He is in all respects, in form and in excellence of mind, if a father may say so, outstanding among citizens. I, therefore, unless you decide otherwise, will come myself and bring my son, with a fifty-oared ship

[1] "holding out" is interpreted by Erotian as "offering help". διαρκεῦντες: βοηθοῦντες Erot. 34. 20N.

412 πληρώσας τοῖσιν | ἐμοῖσι τέλεσιν ὑπηρεσίας τε ἰητρικὰς καὶ πολεμικάς, ἵνα ἐς ἀμφότερα βοηθῶμεν. ὁ μὲν εἶπε, τοῖσι δὲ ἔδοξεν, οἱ δὲ ἀπεστάλησαν.

4. Συνέβησε δὲ ὁ Νεβρὸς οὗτος καὶ Καλυδώνιον ἄνδρα παρ' ἑωυτῷ τρεφόμενον, ὑπὲρ οὗ τὸ αὐτίκα ὁ λόγος δηλώσει, ὅταν ἡ χρῆσις ἔλθῃ. ὅτε δ' οὖν ἀφίκοντο οὗτοι οἱ ἄνδρες οὗ τὸ στρατόπεδον ἐπετελεῖτο, ὁ θεὸς ἔχαιρεν· οἵ τε γὰρ θάνατοι τῶν στρατιωτῶν ἔληξαν, καὶ θείῃ τύχῃ ἵππου τοῦ Εὐρυλόχου, ὃς ἡγεῖτο τοῦ πολέμου Θεσσαλὸς ἐὼν καὶ ἄνωθεν ἐξ Ἡρακλειδῶν, κρούσαντος τὸν σωλῆνα τῇ ὁπλῇ, δι' οὗ τὸ ὕδωρ ἤγετο ἐς τὸ τεῖχος, ὁκότε διακονίεσθαι ἤθελεν, Νεβρὸς φαρμάκοισιν ἐμίηνε τὸ ὕδωρ· ἔνθεν αἱ κοιλίαι τῶν Κρισαίων ἐφθάρησαν, καὶ μεγάλα δή τι ξυνεβάλετο πρὸς τὸ ἁλῶναι τὴν πόλιν· καὶ ἐντεῦθεν αἱ γνῶμαι ἐπήρθησαν τῶν πολιορκεόντων, ὡς τοῦ θεοῦ ἐπικουρέοντος ἤδη σαφῶς. προσβολὰς δὲ ποιευμένων καὶ ἆθλα προτιθέντων τοῖσι πρώτοισιν ἐπὶ τὸ τεῖχος. ἀναβάσιος ὁ ἀγὼν ἦν καρτερώτατος, καὶ ἡ πόλις ᾑρεῖτο· ἀνέβη πρῶτος ἐπὶ τὸ τεῖχος Χρύσος καὶ κατέλαβε τὸν πύργον, ξυνείπετο δὲ αὐτῷ ἐκ ποδὸς ξυνασπίζων ὁ ἀνὴρ ὁ Καλυδώνιος, περὶ οὗ ἔλεξα. ὁ μὲν Χρύσος δόρατι πληγεὶς ἔπεσε κατ' ἄκρης ἐκ τοῦ πύργου ὑπὸ Μερμοδέω, τοῦ Λύκου δὲ ἀδελφεοῦ, ὃς ἀπέθανε λευστὸς ὅτε ἦλθεν ἐς τὸ ἄδυτον τὸν τρίποδα συλήσων. ἡ δ' οὖν πόλις οὕτως ἥλω· ἥ τε τοῦ Νεβροῦ ἐπικουρίη σὺν Χρύσῳ ὀρθῶς ἀπήντησε καὶ κατὰ τὰ ἰατρικὰ καὶ κατὰ τὰ πολεμικά, ὅ τε θεὸς ἠλήθευσε, καὶ ἃ ὑπέσχετο ἐποίησεν. ἐφ' οἷσιν οἱ Ἀμφικτύονες τῷ μὲν Ἀπόλλωνι νηὸν ἀνέθεσαν, τὸν νῦν ἐόντα ἐν Δελφοῖσιν, ἀγῶνά τε γυμνικὸν καὶ ἱππικὸν πρότερον οὐ τιθέντες νῦν τιθέασι, τήν τε τῶν
414 Κρισαίων χώρην ἅπασαν καθιέρωσαν, | τῷ δόντι ἃ ἔδωκε διδόντες καθ' ὅτι ἔχρησε, τόν τε τοῦ Νεβροῦ παῖδα Χρύσον ἔθαψαν ἐν τῷ ἱπποδρόμῳ, καὶ ξυνέταξαν δημοσίῃ Δελφοὺς ἐναγίζειν· Ἀσκληπιάδῃσιν δὲ τοῖσιν ἐκ Κῶ ἐδόθη Νεβροῦ χάριτι προμυθίη πρὸς μαντείην, καθάπερ τοῖσιν ἱερομνήμοσι, Καλυδωνίοισι δὲ ἀπ' ἐκείνου τοῦ ἀνδρὸς καὶ ἐκείνης τῆς ὑπουργίης καὶ νῦν ἐν Δελφοῖσι προμαντείη καὶ αἰεισιτίη δέδοται. ἀλλ' ἐπάνειμι ἐπὶ τὰ ἡμέτερα· ὅτι γὰρ ἀληθέα λέγω, τοῦ πατρὸς καὶ ἐμεῦ ἐπελθόντων, Ἀμφικτύονες ἀνενεώσαντο ταῦτα καὶ ἀπέδοσαν, καὶ ἐν στήλῃ ἀναγράψαντες ἐν Δελφοῖσιν ἀνέθεσαν. καὶ τούτου μέν μοι τοῦ λόγου τέλος, ἐνταῦθα καθαρῶς δείκνυσι τοὺς ἡμετέρους προγόνους ὑμέων εὐεργέτας.

5. Τοῦτον δὲ καταθέμενος, ἄλλον αἱρήσομαι περὶ τῶν αὐτῶν, οὐ τὸν αὐτόν· ὅτε γὰρ βασιλεὺς ὁ μέγας ξὺν Πέρσῃσιν καὶ τοῖσιν ἄλλοισι βαρβάροισιν ἐστράτευσεν ἐπὶ τοὺς μὴ διδόντας ὕδωρ καὶ γῆν Ἑλλήνων, ἡ

---

1 τελέσμασιν U ‖ 4 συνενέβησε VHI ‖ 15 ἀναβάσιος: scripsi ἀναβασίημος VHI ἀναβάσιμος U ‖ 17 προέλεξα UHI ‖ 18 κατάκρις U ‖ 19 ἔλευστὸς UHI ἐλευστός V correxi ‖ 20 ἤ το U ἡ δ' HI ‖ 25 καθιερώσαντο UHI ‖ 28 προμήθεια U προμηθία V προμυθίη H προμηθίη I ‖ 30 ἐν Δελφοῖσι: ἀδελφοῖς U προμαντεία U προμαντίη V διισιτίη U διεισιτίη VHI ‖ 31 ἐμεῦν V λέγω καὶ ἐμεῦν (om. τοῦ πατρος) I ‖ 33 ἀνέθησαν U ‖ 36 τούτων U

equipped at my expense with medical and military assistance so that we can give aid in both." So he spoke. The Coans agreed and they were dispatched.

4. This Fawn brought on board with him a Calydonian man who had been raised with him, about whom my story will soon speak when the need arises. When, then, these men came to where the army was deployed, the god was delighted, for the deaths of the soldiers ceased, and when by divine chance, while the horse of Eurylochus (who commanded the army, being a Thessalian and descended from the Heraclids) when he was rolling in the dust, broke through the pipe with his hoof where the water was led towards the wall, Fawn polluted the water with drugs. Thereupon the intestines of the Criseans were ruined, and it contributed a great deal to the capture of the city. From then on, the spirits of the besiegers were elevated in the belief that the god was clearly giving aid. They launched attacks; they set up prizes for those first onto the walls; the contest to mount the wall became very strong, and the city was taken. Gold was first to mount the wall and he captured the tower. With him, on foot and carrying his shield, went the man from Calydon of whom I spoke. Gold fell from the top of the tower, struck by a spear thrown by Mermodeus, brother of Wolf (Lycus), who perished by stoning when he entered the inner sanctum to loot the tripod. So, the city was taken in this way. The assistance of Fawn with Gold in medical and military matters properly came to pass. And the god proved true and did what he promised. For that the Amphictyons dedicated a temple to Apollo, the one which is now at Delphi, and never before having established athletic and equestrian contests, they now established them, and they sanctified the entire land of the Criseans, giving to the giver what he had given, as he prophesied. Fawn's son Gold they buried in the hippodrome and instructed the Delphians to offer sacrifice to him at public expense. And to the Asclepiads from Cos was given, for Fawn's sake, the right of priority in consulting the oracle, the same as the Hieromnemones[1], and to the Calydonians on account of that man and his service even now has been given priority in consultation at Delphi and perpetual rights to food. But I proceed to our situation. Because what I am saying is true, when my father and I went there the Amphictyons renewed those things and granted them to us, and they inscribed it on a column which they set up at Delphi. And the end of this story is that in that place it demonstrates in all simplicity that our ancestors were your benefactors.

5. I shall lay down that story and pick up another, a different one about the same things. When the Great King with the Persians and other barbarians made war on those Greeks who did not give him earth and water, our country chose

[1] Hieromnemones was the name of religious and administrative officials in many Greek states. The Delphic Amphictyony had hieromnemones as representatives from member states, whose functions are described in the inscription IG II^2 1126.

πατρὶς ἡ ἡμετέρη εἵλετο μᾶλλον πανδημεὶ ἀπολέσθαι, ὡς μὴ καθ' ὑμέων τε καὶ τῶν ταὐτὰ ὑμῖν γινωσκόντων ὅπλα πολέμια λάβῃ καὶ ἐν νεῦσι στρατείην ἀποστείλῃ, ἀλλ' ἀνένευσε καλόν τι καὶ ἄξιον τῶν πατέρων μεγαλοφρονευμένη, οἳ λέγονται γηγενεῖς τε εἶναι καὶ Ἡρακλεῖδαι. ἔδοξεν οὖν σφιν, τεσσάρων ἐόντων τειχέων ἐν τῇ νήσῳ, πάντ' ἐκλιπεῖν καὶ ἐς τὰ ὄρεα καταφυγοῦσιν ἀντέχεσθαι σωτηρίης. ὅθεν δὴ τί κακὸν οὐκ ἀπήντησε; χώρης λεηλατεομένης καὶ σωμάτων ἐλευθέρων ἀνδραποδιζομένων καὶ κτεινομένων ἐχθρῶν νόμῳ, τῆς δὲ πόλιος καὶ τῶν ἄλλων ἐρυμάτων καὶ ἱερῶν καταιθαλουμένων, ἔτι δὲ καὶ τῇ θυγατρὶ
416 τοῦ Λυγδάμιος Ἀρτεμισίῃ κατὰ πατρῷον | νεῖκος δοθέντων ἐκσαγηνεῦσαι πάντα ὅσα λοιπὰ ἦν. ἀλλὰ γάρ, ὡς ἔοικε, θεοῖσιν οὐκ ἠμελεύμεθα· χειμώνων δὲ γενομένων ἐξαισίων, αἵ τε νῆες τῆς Ἀρτεμισίης ἐκινδύνευσαν ἅπασαι ἀπολέσθαι, πολλαὶ δὲ καὶ ἀπώλοντο, ἔς τε τὸ στράτευμα αὐτῆς πολλοὶ κεραυνοὶ ἐνέπεσον, σπάνιόν τι τῆς νήσου κεραυνουμένης· λέγεται δὲ καὶ φάσματα ἡρώων τῇ γυναικὶ ὀφθῆναι· ἃ δὴ πάντα φοβηθεῖσα ἀπέστη ἔργων ἀνηκέστων, ὁμολογίην πικρὴν ποιησαμένη, καὶ λίην πικρὴν λέγεσθαι, ὥστε ἀφείσθω. ἀποδώσω δὲ καὶ ἐνταῦθα προγόνοισι τοῖσιν ἐμοῖσι κυριότητα οὐ ψευδέα τοῦ μήτ' ἐφ' ὑμέας, μήτ' ἐπὶ Λακεδαιμονίους ἤ τινας ἄλλους Ἑλλήνων, Κῴους ἑκούσια ὅπλα λαβεῖν, καίπερ πολλῶν τῶν ὁμοῦ νήσους τε καὶ Ἀσίην οἰκεόντων συναψαμένων τοῖσι βαρβάροισι τοῦ πολέμου οὐ βίῃ.

6. Οἱ γὰρ προεστῶτες τότε τῆς πόλιος ἦσαν Κάδμος τε καὶ Ἱππόλοχος· ἐπ' ἀληθεῖ δὲ κεῖται προγόνους ἐμοὺς εἶναι τόν τε Κάδμον καὶ τὸν Ἱππόλοχον· ὁ μὲν γὰρ Κάδμος, ὃς καὶ τὴν βουλὴν αὐτὴν ἤρτυσεν, ἔστι τῆς ἐμῆς μητρός, ὁ δ' Ἱππόλοχος ἐξ Ἀσκληπιαδέων τέταρτος ἀπὸ Νέβρου τοῦ Κρισαίους συγκαθελόντος, ἡμεῖς δ' Ἀσκληπιάδαι κατ' ἀνδρογένειαν· ὥστε καὶ τοῦτο τὸ καλὸν τῶν ἡμετέρων προγόνων προελέσθαι. ἐπάνειμι δ' ἐπὶ τὸν Κάδμον· οὗτος γὰρ δὴ ὁ ἀνὴρ οὕτως ἔσπευδε τὰ τῶν Ἑλλήνων καλὰ ὥστε, ὁκότε ἔληξεν ἡ χώρη πολιορκεομένη ὑπὸ Ἀρτεμισίης, αὐτοῦ καταλιπὼν τὴν γυναῖκα καὶ γενεήν, ᾤχετο ξὺν τοῖσι ταῦτα αἱρεομένοισιν ἐπὶ Σικελίης, ὅκως Γέλωνα καὶ τοὺς ἀδελφοὺς κωλύσει φιλίην ξυνθέσθαι κατὰ Ἑλλήνων πρὸς τοὺς βαρβάρους· διεπρήξατο δὲ καὶ ἄλλα πολλὰ καλὰ ἔργα, ἃ μηκύνειν οὐ πρόσκαιρον. αἱ μὲν δὴ δημόσιαι
418 καὶ ἡμέων προγόνων ὑπουργίαι ἐς ὑμέας | καὶ τοὺς ἄλλους Ἕλληνας αὗται καὶ τοιαῦται πολλαί· καὶ γὰρ ἐκλείπει ἡ δύναμις τοῦ λόγου.

7. Ἔρχομαι δ' ἤδη ἐνειδόσιν εὐεργεσίην Ἱπποκράτους πατρὸς ἐμέο προέχεσθαι· λέγων δ' ἂν ἀληθεύοιμι οὕτως· ὁκότε λοιμοῦ ῥέοντος διὰ τῆς

---

2 πολέμια: πρὸ δὲ μία VHI || 5 σφιν: αὐτοῖς U || 6 δήτι κακô U δήτι κακῶν VHI corr. Asul. || 7 δὲ ἠλατευομένης VHI δὲ ἠλατευμένης U corr. Com. || 8 ἐκτεινομένων U ἐχθρῷ UI || 10 λυγμάλιος U νῖκος V νίκος U νῖκος H I non legibilem corr. Li. ἐκσαγήνευσε V || 14 ἐνέπεσον UHI || 19 ἤ τινας: scripsi ἑτέρους mss. || 26 κρισαίου U κρισσαίου V κρισαίους ms. K(Li.)Com. || 30 ταῦτα: τὰ αὐτά UIH || 36 ἔρχωμαι U ἐνειδαισιν V ἐν εἴδεσιν HI ἐνειδόσιν U || 37 ἢ προσεύχεσθαι U ἢ προέχεσθαι V προέχεσθαι (om. ἢ): HI

rather to perish all together so as not to take up arms and set out in a naval expedition against you and those that agreed with you. In this refusal the Coans exhibited a greatness of mind worthy of our forefathers, who are said to be earth born and Heraclids. They decided, though there were four fortified towns on the island, to abandon them all, and to take flight to the mountains and there to cling to their salvation. And from this what evil did not come to pass? Their land was devastated, their free persons were enslaved and killed by the law of enemies, the city and all other defenses, and the sacred places were burned, and finally they were given over to Artemisia, daughter of Lygdamis, in accordance with an ancestral quarrel, to catch with a dragnet everything that was left. Still, it seems, we were not neglected by the gods. There were extraordinary storms and the ships of Artemisia were all in danger of destruction. Many were destroyed and many thunderbolts fell on her army, but the island was hardly touched by lightning. And it is said that visions of heroes were seen by the woman. And terrified at all this she departed with her work undone, having made a bitter agreement, too bitter to describe, so let it go. But I will here give to my ancestors the dignity, no false one, that the Coans never took up willing arms against you, nor against the Lacedemonians nor any other Greeks, though many of the surrounding people who lived on the islands and mainland of Asia joined with the barbarians in the war when they were not forced.

6. Cadmus and Hippolochus were at that time in charge of the city. And it is in the realm of truth that Cadmus and Hippolochus are my forebears. Cadmus who formed the plan itself is in the line of my mother, and Hippolochus is an Asclepiad, fourth in line from Fawn, who destroyed the Criseans. And we are Asclepiads by male descent. Therefore, it was some of our ancestors who undertook this excellent work also. I proceed to Cadmus, who was so concerned that the Greeks' affairs should prosper, that when the country was no longer besieged by Artemisia he left his wife and family behind and went with the rest who had made this choice to Sicily, trying to prevent Gelon and his brothers from making a treaty of friendship with the barbarians against the Greeks.[1] He did many other fine deeds as well, on which there is not time to elaborate. The benefits to you and to the rest of Greece from my city and my ancestors are these and many others like them. My rhetorical power is not adequate to them.

7. I now proceed to hold forth, for you who are well aware of it, the benefaction of my father Hippocrates, and what I say shall be the truth. In the

[1] Cf. Herodotus 7.163-4, and above, Introduction, p. 3.

βαρβάρου ἣ ὑπέρκειται Ἰλλυριῶν καὶ Παιόνων, ὁκότε δὴ ἐπὶ ταύτην τὴν χώρην ἱκνεῖτο τὸ κακόν, οἱ τούτων τῶν ἐθνέων βασιλῆες κατὰ δόξαν ἰητρικὴν ἣ ἀληθὴς ἐοῦσα πανταχόθι ἴσχυεν ἔρχεσθαι, κατὰ πατρὸς τοῦ ἐμέο πέμπουσιν ἐπὶ Θεσσαλίης, ἐκεῖ γὰρ δὴ ὁ ἐμὸς πατὴρ καὶ πρότερον καὶ νῦν οἴκησιν εἶχε, καλέοντες αὐτὸν ἐς ἐπικουρίην, χρυσοῦ τε καὶ ἀργύρου καὶ ἄλλων κτεάνων οὐ μὴν ἔφασαν πέμψειν ἕξειν, ἀλλὰ καὶ ἀποίσασθαι ὁκόσα ἂν αὐτὸς ἐθέλῃ ἐπαμύναντα. ὁ δὲ ἐρώτησιν ποιησάμενος ὁκοῖαί τινες ἐν μέρει κινήσιες γίνονται κατά τε καύματα καὶ ἀνέμους καὶ ἀχλύας καὶ τἄλλα ἃ πέφυκε ἕξιας κινεῖν παρὰ τὸ καθεστηκός· ὁκότε δὴ πάντων μαθήσιας ἀνείλετο, τοὺς μὲν χωρεῖν ἐκέλευσεν ὀπίσω, ἀποφηνάμενος μὴ οἷός τε εἶναι δύναμιν ἐς χώρην τὴν ἐκείνων ἰέναι· ὅκως δὲ εἶχε ταχέως, αὐτὸς μὲν Θεσσαλοῖσιν ἠρτύετο παραγγέλλειν ὁκοίοισι χρὴ τρόποισι κακοῦ τοῦ προσιόντος εὐλαβείην ποιεῖσθαι, καὶ ξυγγράφων θεραπείην ἐξετίθει περὶ τὰς πόλιας· ἐμὲ δὲ ἐπὶ Μακεδονίης ἐξαπέστειλε, βασιλεῦσι γὰρ Ἡρακλειδέων οἳ ἐκεῖ κατέχουσι πατρικὴ ξεινίη ὑπῆρχεν ἡμῖν. κἀγὼ μὲν ᾖειν ἵνα με ὁ πατὴρ ἐκέλευσεν ἀπὸ Θεσσαλίας ἀρήξων τοῖσιν ἐκεῖ· συνετέτακτο δέ μοι ξυμβαλεῖν ἐς πόλιν τὴν ὑμετέρην. ἀδελφεὸν δὲ τὸν ἐμὸν Δράκοντα ἐκ Παγασέων ὁρμηθέντα πλοῦν ποιεῖσθαι ἐφ' Ἑλλησπόντου ἐκέλευσε, παραπλησίην δοὺς
420 ὑποθήκην ᾗ αὐτὸς ἔπρησσεν· οὐ | γὰρ πάντες τόποι τὰ αὐτὰ φέρουσι παθήματα, διὰ τὸ μὴ πάντῃ τὰ περιέχοντα ἐξ ἀέρος ὅμοια εἶναι. Πολύβιον δὲ τὸν τὴν θυγατέρα ἔχοντα, ἐμὴν δὲ ἀδελφεήν, καὶ ἄλλους τῶν μαθητέων διέπεμπεν ἐς ἑτέρας ἑτέρων καὶ πλωτὰς καὶ ὁδοὺς πορευσομένους, ὅκως ὅτι πλείστοισιν ἐπαρήξαι. ὡς δὲ δὴ τὰ κατὰ Θεσσαλίην ἠνύσατο, ἐπορεύετο τοῖσιν ἐχομένοισιν ἔθνεσι βοηθέων· ἐπὶ Πύλας δὲ ἐλθὼν Δωριεῦσι καὶ τοῖσιν ὁμοῦ Φωκέων ἐπήρκει· καὶ ὁκότε δὴ ἐς Δελφοὺς ἀφίκετο, ὑπὲρ Ἑλλήνων ἱκεσίην ἔθετο τῷ θεῷ, καὶ θύσας ἤνυε τὴν ἐπὶ Βοιωτῶν, τοῖσι δ' ἐκεῖ ἐπαμύνας ἀναλόγως, ἐν τῇ ὑμετέρῃ ἦν, καὶ ἱκανὰ ἃ νῦν ἐγὼ ἐπαγορεύω τὰ ὑμῖν σωτήρια ἐκ θυμοῦ παντὸς εἶπε. δοκέω δ' ὑμέων ὅτι ἀληθεύω πολλοὺς γινώσκειν· οὐ γὰρ πάλαι, ἀλλ' ἔτος ἐστὶ τοῦτο ἔνατον, ἐξ οὗ διελήλυθα καὶ ἐπὶ Πελοπόννησον ἐστελλόμην, καὶ τοῖσιν ἐκείνῃ οἰκέουσι βοηθήσων. πάντοθεν δ' ἡμῖν καὶ λόγῳ καὶ ἔργῳ ἀξίη τιμὴ ἀπήντα, ὥστε μὴ μεταμέλεσθαι ὅτι οὐκ ἠλλαξάμεθα χρηματισμοῦ τοῦ ἐξ Ἰλλυριῶν καὶ Παιόνων. παρὰ δὲ τὰς ἄλλας πόλιας τὰ παρ' ὑμέων δοθέντα μεγάλα ἦν· ἥ τε γὰρ πολιτείη ἡ ὑμετέρη ὑπερῆγε τὰς ἑτέρων· αἱ γὰρ Ἀθῆναι ὑψηλότερόν τι τῶν ἄλλων πόλιων ἐς δόξαν, καὶ ὁ ἐν τῷ ὑμετέρῳ θεητρῳ χρύσεος στέφανος ἐπιτεθεὶς

---

1 πλειόνων mss. corr. Com.   ἐπ' αὐτὴν U ‖ 2 ἵκνετο V ἧκε H ἧκεν I ‖ 3 πανταχόθεν UHI ante κατὰ add. καὶ V ‖ 6 κτεάτων U   οὔ μιν VH   οὐ μὲν I   ἔφασεν U   ἐξῆν U   ἐξ ἦν HI ‖ 7 ἐπαμύναντι U ‖ 9 ἕξιας: ἕξιης V   ὄξεις U om. HI ‖ 10 χώραν U   χώρην HI ‖ 12 deficit ms. I ‖ 13 τόποις U   προιόντι U ‖ 18 ἡμετέρην U ‖ 21 βοηθηματα UH   παντα (om. τὰ) U ‖ 23 διεπεμπ' ἐς V   πλοτὰς UH ‖ 24 παρεσομένους U ‖ 25 βοηθῶν U ‖ 32 ἐκείνην U βοηθήσονται U   βοηθήσοντες V   βοηθήσοντα H corr. Asul. ‖ 34 ἰλλυριοῦ V ‖ 37 χύσεος V

time in which the plague was running through the barbarian land north of the Illyrians and Paeonians, when the evil reached that area, the kings of those peoples sent to Thessaly after my father because of his reputation as a physician, which, being a true one, had managed to go everywhere. He had lived in Thessaly previously and had a dwelling there then. They summoned him to help, saying that they were not going to send gold and silver and other possessions for him to have, but said that he could carry away all that he wanted when he had come to help. And he made inquiry what kinds of disturbances there were, area by area, in heat and winds and mist and other things that produce unusual conditions. When he had gotten everyone's information he told them to go back, pretending that he was unable to go to their country. But as quickly as he could he arranged to announce to the Thessalians by what means they could contrive protection against the evil that was coming, and, writing down the therapy, he posted it around the cities. And he sent me to Macedonia, for we had an ancestral guest-friendship with the kings of the Heraclids who are in power there. And I went where my father ordered me, outside Thessaly, to help the people there. And I was instructed to be of use in your city. But my brother Draco he commanded to set out from Pagasae and sail to the Hellespont, giving him advice similar to that on which he himself had acted. For not all places produce the same diseases because the environment from the air is not alike everywhere. And he sent Polybius, his son-in-law and my brother-in-law, along with others of his students to go travel various waterways and highways of different regions so that he could help as many as possible. When he had finished his business in Thessaly he traveled to neighboring peoples offering help. Going to Pylae he ministered to the Dorians and the nearby Phocians. And when he came to Delphi he made a suppliance to the god in behalf of the Greeks. And having made sacrifice he hurried to the territory of the Boeotians, and having helped them similarly he spent time in your territory, and he spoke the means of your safety, with great feeling, as I shall relate. I believe many of you know that I speak the truth, for it is not long ago, but this is the ninth year since I traveled about and was sent to the Peloponnesus to help also those who lived there. On all sides in word and deed worthy honor came to us, so that we did not regret that we did not get money from the Illyrians and Paeonians. But what was given by you was large compared to other cities, for your city outdid the cities of other peoples. Athens is, after all something higher for reputation, and the gold crown presented in your theater ζήλου πρὸς τὸ ἄκρον ἦγεν. ἀλλὰ καὶ τοῦτο τὸ καλὸν ὑπερεβάλεσθε, μυήσαντες τὰ Δήμητρος καὶ κόρης ὄργια καὶ τὸν πατέρα καὶ ἐμὲ δημοσίῃ.

8. Καὶ τρεῖς μὲν αὗταί μοι οἷον ἀνύοντι ἐξέλκειν τε τοὺς λόγους καὶ
422 σχοινίων προέχεσθαι ⟨αἱ⟩ πόλιός τε καὶ προγόνων καὶ πατρὸς τοῦ ἐμέο χάριτες ξὺν | πολλοῖσιν Ἑλλήνων· τετάρτην δ' ἀναλήψομαι λέγειν ὑπουργίην, ἥν, ὡς ὑπεθέμην, ἐς ὑμᾶς ἐγὼ καὶ ὁ πατὴρ ὁ ἐμὸς κατεθέμεθα. ὅτε γὰρ Ἀλκιβιάδην ⟨ἡ πόλις⟩ ἐξέπεμπεν ἐπὶ Σικελίης πολλῇ μὲν δυνάμει, οὐχ οὕτω δὲ πολλῇ ὡς θαυμαστῇ, εἰ γὰρ ὡς ἔργα, λόγου ἐν ἐκκλησίῃ ὑπὲρ ἰητροῦ προπεσόντος ὃν δέοι ἀκολουθεῖν τῷ στρατεύματι, παρελθὼν ὁ πατὴρ ὑπέσχετο ἐμὲ ἐπὶ τὰ ὑμέτερα σώματα δώσειν, τοῖσιν ἰδίοισι δαπανήμασι κατεσκευασμένον καὶ ἄτερ μισθῶν αἰτήσιος ἕως ἂν ὁ στόλος ἀποδημῇ, ἐν ἐλάσσονι τιθέμενος τὸ λυσιτελὲς ἀξιόχρεων ἐὸν τῆς ὑμῖν χρείης ἐσομένης. ἐγὼ γὰρ οὐχ ὅκως ἂν τὰ ὑπάρχοντα κατεδαπάνουν, ὃ ἐποίεον ὑμῖν ὑπουργέων, ἀλλὰ καὶ ἐν ἄλλοισι μεγάλοισιν ἔργοισιν ἐτετάγμην. καὶ τοῦτο ἐλάχιστον τῶν μελλόντων ῥηθήσεσθαι· προείλετο γὰρ μᾶλλον ὁ πατὴρ ἐν ἐμοὶ τῷ υἱεῖ καὶ ἐν γῇ ὀθνείᾳ ἀλύειν καὶ κατὰ θάλασσαν καὶ κατὰ κινδύνους πολεμικούς, καὶ κατ' ἀρρωστίας, αἳ τοῖσιν ἐν πλανώδεσι βίοισιν εἰθισμέναι εἰσὶ μᾶλλον προσκαθίζειν ἢ τοῖσιν ἐν τεταγμένῃ ζωῇ· ἠπίστατο γὰρ χάριτι χάριτα μετρεῖσθαι, καὶ μὴ οἷόν περ τι ὠνευμένοισιν ἐκ χειρὸς ἐς χεῖρας συναλλάξας ἅπαξ ἀπιέναι. ὁ μὲν δὴ τοιούτων ὑπῆρξεν· ἐγὼ δέ, ἅτε παῖς ἐὼν ἐκείνου, οὐδὲν ἐλλείπω φιλοτιμίης καὶ τέχνης, βοηθέων καὶ κινδυνεύων σὺν ὑμῖν ὁκότε που καιρὸς εἴη· καὶ ἐς ταῦτά με ἀμφότερα οὔτε νοῦσος οὔτε κακοπαθείη οὔτε φόβος ὁ ἐν θαλάσσῃ καὶ ὁ ἐν χέρσῳ πολεμίων εἴργει· μαρτυρίη δὲ οὐκ ἐν ἄλλοισί τισιν, ἐν δ' ὑμῖν αὐτοῖσι
424 κεῖται· ὥστε, εἴ τῳ ἀντιλεκτέον, ἀναστήτω μηδὲν ὀκνήσας, ἀλλ' οὐ δοκέω ψεύδεσθαι. ταῦτα δὲ πρήξας | ἐπὶ τρία ἔτεα, στεφανωθείς τε χρυσέῳ στεφάνῳ, καὶ ἔτι κάλλιον εὐφημεύμενος, ἐς τὴν ἰδίην ἀπῆλθον ἐπὶ γάμον, ὡς διαδόχους καταστήσαιμι καὶ τέχνης καὶ γενεῆς ἡμετέρης.

9. Ἃ μὲν δὴ παρὰ πόλιος, προγόνων, πατρός τε καὶ ἐμέο ὑμῖν ὑπάρχει, ταῦτ' ἐστίν· εἴρηται δὲ καὶ ὧν ἡμεῖς παρ' ὑμέων ἐπαυράμεθα. δοκέω δὲ πολλοὺς ὑμέων θαυμάζειν, ὅτεων χάριν ταῦτα ἀναμεμέτρηται· ὡς οὖν καὶ ὑμεῖς εἰδῆτε καὶ ἐμοὶ γίνηται ἃ ἐγὼ ἐπιθυμέω, καιρὸς λέγειν. ὁ πατήρ, ὦ ἄνδρες Ἀθηναῖοι, καὶ ἐγὼ αἰτεόμεθα ὑμέας, οὕτω γὰρ εἰπεῖν ἐλευθέρους καὶ φίλους παρὰ φίλων τυχεῖν ἐλεύθερον, ἐκ πατρίδος τῆς ὑμετέρης ὅπλα πολέμια μὴ ἄρασθαι· εἰ δὲ δεῖ, ὥσπερ ἴσως δεῖ τοὺς ὑπὲρ τῆς αὐτῶν προεληλυθότας, καὶ δεόμεθα μὴ ἡμέας ἐόντας ἀξιωμάτων

---

2 ante μυστήρια add. ὄργια U ‖ 3 ἀοϊόντι ἐξελκεατοὺς V οἷον ἀνύοντι εξέλκεάτ ε τοὺς U ἂν οἷόν τι ἐξελκεάτε H post λόγους add. καὶ U ‖ 4 προέχεσθε V αἱ scripsi ‖ 7 ἡ πόλις coni. Li. secutus Foës ἐξέπεμψεν H ‖ 8 ἦν γὰρ ὅσ' ἔργα coni. Li. ‖ 9 προσπεσόντος U ‖ 10 ἐμὲ om. U δῶσιν U ‖ 12 ἀποδημοῖ H ἐὼν U ‖ 14 κατεδαπάνων edd. -ουν mss. ‖ 17 ὀθνείᾳ ἀλύειν: scripsi ὀθνείαις ἀλλεύειν V ὀθνεία σαλεύειν U ὀθνείας ἀλεύειν H ante πολεμικούς add. καὶ U ‖ 19 ἐπίστατο U ‖ 22 ἐλλίπω φιλοτίας U ‖ 23 ἡμῖν UV ‖ 24 χερσὶ mss. correxi ‖ 25 δὲ om. H ‖ 27 ἔτεα: ἔτι U ‖ 29 γάρμον U ‖ 31 ἐπαυρώμεθα U ‖ 32 ἀναμετρεῖται V ‖ 33 εἴδηται U ἰδῆτε H γίνεται U ‖ 36 ἄρασθε H δεῖ: δὴ U

took us to the heights of envy. But you even exceeded that elegance by initiating both my father and me into the ceremonies of Demeter and Kore at public expense.

8. These are the three; I have succeeded in pulling forth the arguments without using ropes; the three favors done by my city and my ancestors and my father, for Greeks generally. I shall undertake to describe a fourth benefit which as I suggested, I and my father did for you. When the city was sending Alcibiades to Sicily with a great force, not just great, but amazing (I wish that it had been as amazing as the need!), when there was preliminary discussion in the ecclesia about a physician who was needed to accompany the army, my father came forward and proposed to offer me for the care of your bodies, equipping me by his own expenditure and without request for pay so long as the expedition was away, making light of the expense because it was only appropriate to your coming need. For I would not only have squandered whatever I had, which in fact I did, in helping you, but I was also dispatched in other great actions. And this is a small part of what there is to be said. For my father chose in your behalf, for me his son, that I wander about in a strange land, and on the sea, and in the dangers of war, and among sicknesses, which generally settle more on those whose lives are spent wandering about than on those in a settled life. For he knew that one measures a favor by a favor, and does not, as with items of commerce, once and for all pass it from hand to hand and go away. So, he initiated these things. I, being his child, was not behind in desire for honor and in the science; I helped you and underwent dangers whenever the time came. And in both of those pursuits not disease nor distress nor fear of the enemy on the sea or land held me back. The witness of that lies in no others than you yourselves. Wherefore, if someone needs to contradict me let him stand forth without hesitation. But I do not expect to be proved false. Having done these things for three years, having been crowned with a golden crown and praised yet more decorously, I went home to my own land to marry, so that I could produce successors for our science and our family line.

9. These, then, are the things that came to you from my city, my ancestors, my father, and myself. And I have described what we got in return from you. I expect that many of you are wondering for what reason I have been measuring these things out. So that you can know, and so that I can achieve what I want, it is time to say it. My father and I, oh men of Athens, beseech you (for, for free men to speak so, and for friends to get favors from friends is the behavior of free men) do not raise up aggressive war from your land. And if it is necessary, as it is perhaps for those who have gone forth in behalf of their own land, we beg that

μεγάλων, καὶ τοιούτων προϋπάρξαντας, ἐν δούλων μέρει τιθήσεσθαι· ἔτι δέ, καὶ γὰρ οὕτως ἁρμόσει λέγειν, μὴ ποιήσησθε, ἱκετεύομεν, τὰ ἡμέτερα ὑμῖν αὐτοῖσι δουρίκτητα πολλοὶ μειόνων ἣν ἐπάνω γένησθε, ἀλλ' ὑπίδεσθε καὶ τοῦτο ὅτι ἑτέρως ἕτερα ἡ τύχη ταχύνει· καί ποτε σμικρῶν μεγάλοι προεδεήθησαν, καὶ οἱ καρτεροὶ δι' ἀσθενέας σωτηρίης ἔτυχον. δοκέω δὲ σύνδηλον, ὡς μὴ ἐνδηλότερον εἴπω, ὅτι ἐφ' ἑνὶ ἀνδρὶ οὐ πόλις, ἀλλὰ πολλὰ ἔθνεα ἤδη ποτὲ ὤφθη ὠφεληθέντα ἐν πολεμικοῖσι, καὶ ἔνθα τέχνη ἰσχύει. μηδὲ ἡμέας ἀποβάλησθε· καὶ γὰρ οὐδὲ ἀπόβλητοι ἐσμέν, ὡς ἐν ὑμῖν μαρτυρίη κεῖται· ἀλλ' ἀρχὴν μὲν οἱ θεοί, ἔνθεν γένος εὔχομαι εἶναι, Ἀσκληπιὸς καὶ Ἡρακλῆς, ἐπ' ὠφελείῃ ἀνθρώπων ἐγένοντο, καὶ τούτους δι' ἀρετὴν τὴν ἐνταῦθα ἐν θεῶν χώρῃ ἔχουσι πάντες· πόλις δὲ ἐμὴ καὶ ἐγὼ ὁ λέγων ἐς τοιούτους ἀνερχόμεθα, ὡς ἀνθρώπων λόγοι κατέχουσιν· ὅθεν δὴ καὶ ὑπὲρ Ἑλλήνων φανεύμεθα ἀμφότεροι ταύτῃ
426 προϊστάμενοι καὶ ἐπὶ παντὶ καλλίστῳ· οὐ γὰρ μῦθος | τὰ Τρωϊκὰ ἀλλ' ἔργα, ἐν οἷσιν ἡ Κῶς σὺν τῇσιν ἑωυτῆς νήυσιν οὐ πολλοστή, μεγίστη δ' ἐς συμμαχίην ἐστίν· οὕτως δὲ καὶ Ἀσκληπιοῦ παῖδες οὐ τέχνῃ μόνον, ἀλλὰ καὶ ὅπλοισιν ἐπήρκεσαν Ἕλλησι· Μαχάων γέ τοι ψυχὴν κατέθετο ἐν τῇ Τρωάδι, ὅτε, ὡς οἱ ταῦτα γράφοντες λέγουσιν, ἐξ ἵππου ἐς πόλιν τὴν Πριάμου ἐσῆλθε. μὴ δὴ μήτε καθότι ἔμφυλοι, μήτε καθότι ἐξ ἐπαρηγόντων ἐπαρήγοντες γεγόναμεν Ἕλλησιν, ἀδικήσητε ἡμέας.

10. Οὐ μηκυνέω οὐδὲ τὰ Κρισαῖα αὖτις οὔτε τὰ Περσικὰ λέγων, ὁκότε καὶ ἀκηκόατε καὶ ἐν χερσὶ μᾶλλον τῶν ἀρτίως εἰρημένων ἐστίν· ἐν θυμῷ δὲ λάβετε καὶ οὕτως εὐεργέτας μὴ ὅσιον ἀδικεῖν. ἡμεῖς δὲ εὐεργέται ὡς τὰ ἔργα φησί. τίνες φανεῖσθε, οἱ πατέρων γεγῶτες οἵων οἱ μυθολόγοι εἶπον, ἂν τὸ ἀδικεῖν ἀντὶ τοῦ χρηστοὶ εἶναι αἱρῆσθε; οὐ γὰρ ἐθέλω πικρότερον λέγειν· κεῖνοι γάρ, ὦ ἄνδρες Ἀθηναῖοι, Ἡρακλείδῃσιν μὲν ἔτινον χάριτας, ἑτέροισι δὲ πολλοῖσιν εὐεργετηθέντες ἐπήρκεσαν· ὑπολίποι δ' ἄν με ἡμέρη μακρὰ λέγοντα, εἰ διεξίοιμι ὁκόσοισιν ὁκόσα ἀπήντηκεν ἀγαθὰ οὐδὲν ἐν χρείῃ ὑμῖν ἐγγεγονόσι. περιβλέψατε δὲ ἑωυτοὺς καὶ μηδὲ ἐμεῦ εἰπόντος γνῶτε ὁκοῖα πρήσσετε· κακὸν ἐξουσίη, ὦ ἄνδρες Ἀθηναῖοι, οὐ γὰρ ἐπίσταται τὰ ἑωυτῆς μέτρῳ ταμιεύεσθαι, ἀλλὰ δή τινας καὶ πόλιας καὶ ἔθνεα ἐλυμήνατο. ἐς ἑτέρους δὲ οἷον ἐς κάτοπτρον βλέψαντες ἴδετε αὐτοὶ ἃ ποιεῖτε, καὶ ἐγὼ ἀληθέα λέγω. καὶ νέος δὲ νόμος ὅστις εὐτυχίῃ πεποιθώς, μὴ καὶ ἐς τὰ δυσπετέα βλέπει· οὐχ ὑμέτερον· πολλὰ γὰρ καὶ ὧδε δαίμονος πεπείρησθε. οὐδὲν ὑμᾶς ἀδικέομεν· εἰ δὲ καὶ

---

2 ὑμέτερα mss. corr. Asul. ex ms. G ‖ 3 πολλοὶ: πολὺ UH γενήσεσθε mss. correxi ‖ ‖ 4 ὑπείδεσθε UV τύχη: ἀρχὴ H ‖ 5 προεδέθησαν VH (deficit hic H, utar ms. G pro trad. Marciani) ‖ 9-10 εὔχομαι θεῖναι U εὐχομεθ' εἶναι G ‖ 11 ἀρετῆς τῆς UG ‖ 15 ἐν οἷσιν G ἐνοιειν V ἐν οἷς U τῇσιν ἑωυτῇσι νήσοισιν V ταῖς ἑωυτῇσι νήσοις U τοῖσιν ἑωυτοῖσι νήσοισιν G ἑωυτῆς Peterson νήυσιν: scripsi πολλόστην μεγίστην VG ‖ 19 ἔμφυλοι μήτε καθότι om. U ‖ 20 ἀδικήσηται U ‖ 21 οὐδὲ: δὲ UG κρίσαιων U ‖ 23 ὑμεῖς δὲ U ὑμέας δὲ V correxi ‖ 24 οἱ…γεγῶτες: τινὲς θεοὶ πατέρων γεγότες U γεγονότες G ‖ 25 αἱρεῖσθαι U ‖ 26 μικρότερον U ‖ 28 με om. U με ἡ G λεγέοντας V λέγοντας U διέξοιμι V ‖ 31 τὰ om. U ‖ 32 ἐμμήνατο U ‖ 34 βλέπεις U βλέπειν V βλέπει Lind. ‖ 35 πεπειρᾶσθαι U

you not put us in the condition of slaves, us who are worthy of so much, and who have been the source of such things as we have. And further, and this will be a fitting way to speak, we beseech you, do not make our possessions your booty, if you who are many prove superior to us lesser numbers, but look on this fact, that fate speeds one thing one way and another another way. Sometimes the great have had need of the small, and the strong have found safety by means of the weak. I think it is clear, and I need not be more clear, that by a single man not just cities, but many nations, have been seen to be helped before this in military affairs, and wherever science is powerful. Do not cast us away. We are not worthy to be cast away, as you yourselves have witnessed. In the beginning, the gods, from whom I claim our race comes, Asclepius and Heracles, were of great benefit to men, and all hold them in the place of gods for their virtue here. And my city, and I, its speaker, go back to them, as the stories of men hold. So it is that we both clearly stand here for the benefit of Greece and in the fairest light. The Trojan War is not a myth, but a fact, and in it Cos with her own ships was not quantitatively great but was very great for the alliance. And thus Asclepius' sons helped the Greeks not by science alone, but by arms. Machaon laid down his life in the Troad when, as those who wrote of it say, he went into Priam's city out of the horse. Do not, because we are of your own people, because we are your benefactors and descended from your benefactors, do not wrong us.

10. I will not stretch this out by speaking at length again about the Crisean affair, nor the Persian War, when you have heard and have it in hand more so than what I have just said. But take it to your hearts that it is not pious to wrong those who have done you good. And we are benefactors, as the facts relate. What will you seem to be, you who descended from such ancestors as the storytellers relate, if you choose to wrong us instead of being good men? I do not wish to say still more bitter words. Your ancestors, oh Athenians, paid back kindness to the sons of Heracles, and gave assistance to many others from whom they had received benefits. A long day would fail me while I was still speaking if I should go through how many good deeds you have done for how many people who had not been of service to you. Look about at yourselves, and recognize, without my saying it, what you are doing. Power is an evil thing, oh men of Athens, because it does not know how to regulate its affairs in a measured way, but it has sullied cities and nations. Look at others as if into a mirror and see what you are doing. And I am telling the truth. It is a youthful ordinance that, having put its faith in success, does not look also at the bad consequences. That is not your way, for you have had much experience of fate in that manner. We are not wronging you. But even if we are doing wrong, let us

ἀδικέομεν, μὴ ὅπλοισιν, ἀλλὰ λόγῳ, κριθῶμεν. παραιτέομαι δὲ ὑμέας καὶ τοῦτο, μὴ ποιῆσαι χάριν ἑτέροισιν ὀφειλῆσαι, ἐπικουρήσασιν ἡμῖν· ἐπικουρήσουσι γάρ, ἢν ὀρθῶς ποιέωσιν, οἵ τε ἐντὸς Θεσσαλίης, Ἄργεος,
428 Λακεδαίμονος, | Μακεδονίης βασιλεῖς, εἴ κου ἕτεροι Ἡρακλεῖδαι ἢ Ἡρακλειδέων συγγενέες οἰκέουσι. κρεῖσσον ἄτερ βίης τὰ δίκαια ποιεῖν ἢ βιασθέντας· οὐκ εἶπον δ' ἐπανάστασιν· τοῦτο δὲ φανερὸν ποιέων, ὅτι πολλοῖσι μελόμεθα ἢ μελησόμεθα, εἰ μὴ πανταχόθεν οἴχεται τὸ χρηστοὺς ἀνθρώπους ἔτι εἶναι. ἐγὼ μὲν οὖν, μικρὴ γάρ μοι δύναμις λόγου, ἅτε πρὸς ἑτέρων ἐπιμέλειαν ἡρμοσμένῳ, ἐνταῦθα καταπαύσω. ἀξιῶ δὲ πρὸς προξένους ὑμετέρους καὶ τοὺς ὑμῖν συμβούλους εἰθισμένους εἶναι, καὶ θεῶν καὶ ἡρώων εἵνεκα καὶ χαρίτων, αἳ ἀνθρώποισι παρ' ἀνθρώπων γίνονται, ἔχθρας μὲν εἴργειν τὰς ἀλλήλων ὑμέας, ἐς δὲ φίλα προτρέπεσθαι· εἰ γὰρ μὴ ἐν τῇ ὑμετέρῃ πόλει τούτων ἐπιτευξόμεθα, οὐκ οἶδ' ὅκου ἐλθόντες ὧν ἱμείρομεν εὐμοιρήσομεν.

---

2 ὑμῖν UV || 3 Αργαῖος V || 6 ἐπαναστᾶσι VG ἐπαναστάσι U || 10 προξένους scripsi ξένους mss. edd. (cf. Nachmanson, *Erotianstud.* 441) || 12 ἔχθραι G ἡμέας VG ἡμᾶς U corr. Asul. || 14 ἐγκυρήσομεν UG

arrive at judgment by reason, not by weapons. I beg this of you also, do not make us incur an obligation to others for assisting us. For others will help us if they behave properly: people in Thessaly, Argos, Sparta, the Macedonian kings, wherever other Heraclids or connections of the Heraclids live. It is better to do what is right without constraint than under force. And I did not say rebellion, but I am making this clear, that many people care or will care about us unless the existence of good men ends everywhere. My power of speech is small, since I have adapted myself to concern for other things, and so I shall stop at this point. But I ask, in the name of those of you who are proxenoi,[1] and those who are used to giving you counsel, and for the sake of the gods and heroes, and the charity that humans give to one another, restrain one another's enmity, and turn it towards friendly acts. If we shall not encounter such things in your city I do not know where we can go to get those good things that we desire.

---

[1]proxenoi: citizens of Athens (similarly in other cities) who represented the interests of foreign states to the governing bodies. The explanation of this word appears in Erotian, and was restored to the text in this place by Nachmanson.

BIBLIOGRAPHY

Artemidori Daldiani onirocriticon libri v, ed., Roger Pack. Leipzig, Teubner: 1963.

Artemidorus, *The Interpretation of Dreams*, tr. Robt. J. White. Park Ridge, N.J.:1975.

Attridge, Harold W. *First Century Cynicism in the Epistles of Heraclitus*. Scholars Press, Missoula, Montana: 1976.

Bean, G.E., and I. M. Cook, "A Walking Tour," *Annual of the British School at Athens* 52 (1957) 119-127.

Benedum, Jost. "Griechische Artztinschriften," ZPE 25 (1977) 265-276.

Bentley, Richard. *A dissertation upon the epistles of Phalaris, Themistocles, Socrates, Euripides, and others, and the fables of Aesop*. London: 1697.

Boissonade, J.F. *Anecdota Graeca III*. Paris 1831.

Bousquet, Jean. "Inscriptions de Delphes." *BCH* 80 (1956) 579-593.

Buck, Carl Darling. *The Greek Dialects*. Chicago: 1955.

Byl, Simon. "Les recentiores du traité pseudo-hippocratique Du *Régime*; quelques problèmes," *Hippocratica, Actes du Colloque Hippocratique de Paris*, ed. M. Grmek (Paris 1980) 73-83.

Casson, Lionel. *Ships and Seamanship in the Ancient World*. Princeton: 1971.

Cohn-Haft, Louis. *The Public Physicians of Ancient Greece*. Northhampton, Mass.: 1956.

Deichgräber, Kurt. *Die griechische Empirikerschule*, 2nd. ed. Berlin: 1965.

De Ley, Herman. "De Samenstelling van de Pseudo-Hippokratische Brievenverzameling en haar plaats in de Traditie." *Handelingen 23 der Koninklijke Zuidnederlandse Maatschappij voor Taal- en Letterkunde en Geschiendenis*. Utrecht: 1969, 45-80.

Diels, Hermann. "Hippokratische Forschungen V. Eine neue Fassung der xix. Hippokratesbriefes." *Hermes* 53 (1918) 57-87.

__ , and Kranz, W. *Die fragmente der Vorsokratiker*. 10th ed., Berlin: 1961.

__ , *Die Handschriften der antiken Ärzte*. Abh. der Konig. preuss. Akad. der Wiss., phil.-hist. Kl., 3. Berlin: 1905.

Diller, Hans. "Die sogennante zweite Fassung des 19. Hippokratesbriefes," *Quellen und Studien zur Geschichte der Naturwissenschaften und der Medizin* III.4 (1933) 35-44.

Dittenberger, William. *Sylloge Inscriptionum Graecarum*³. Berlin: 1915 (repr. Hildesheim: 1960).

Dudley, D. R., *A History of Cynicism*. London: 1937.

Düring, Ingemar. *Chion of Heraclea*. Göteborg: 1951.

Edelstein, Ludwig. "Hippokrates." RE Suppl. 6 (1935) 1290-1346.

__ , *The Hippocratic Oath*, BHM Suppl. 1. Baltimore: 1943, rep. in *Ancient Medicine*, ed. by O. Temkin and C. L. Temkin (Baltimore: 1967) 3-63.

Ehrenberg, Victor, *The Greek State*². London: 1969.

Ermerins, Francis. *Hippocratis et aliorum medicorum veterum reliquiae*. Vol. III, Utrecht: 1860.

Fraser, Peter M. *Ptolemaic Alexandria*. 2 vols. Oxford: 1972.

Galen, Claudii Galeni opera omnia, ed. C. G. Kühn. Leipzig: 1821-30.
__, *Claudii Galeni Pergameni scripta minora*, vols. 1-3, ed. J. Marquardt, I. Müller, and G. Helmreich. Leipzig: 1884-93.
__, *Comm. in Hipp. Epid. III*, ed. Ernst Wenkebach. CMG V 10, 2,1. Berlin: 1936.
__, *Comm. in Hipp. Epid. VI*, ed., Ernst Wenkebach, Franz Pfaff. CMG V 10, 2,2. Berlin: 1940.
__, *Galen on Anatomical Procedures*. Trans. Charles Singer. London: 1956.
Gösswein, Hans-Ulrich. *Die Briefe des Euripides*. Meisenheim am Glan: 1975.
Grmek, Mirko D. (ed.). *Hippocratica. Actes du colloque hippocratique de Paris* (4-9 septembre 1978). Paris: 1980.
Gow, A. S. F. *Machaon*. Cambridge: 1965. (Cambridge Classical Texts and Commentaries).
Hanson, Ann Ellis. *Collectanea Papyrologica*, part 1. Bonn: 1976.
__, "Papyri of Medical Content," Yale Classical Studies 28 (1985) 25-47.
Heinimann, Felix. "Diokles von Karystos und der prophylaktische Brief an König Antigonos," *Museum Helveticum* 12 (1955) 158-172.
Hercher, Rudolf. *Epistolographi graeci*. Paris: 1871.
__, Aelianus. Leipzig: 1866.
Herzog, Rudolph. *Heilige Gesetze von Kos*. Berlin: 1928.
__, *Koische Forschungen und Funde*. Leipzig: 1899.
Hippocrates. *Oeuvres complètes d'Hippocrate.*, ed., Emil Littré. Paris : 1839-1861.
__, *Hippocratis opera quae feruntur omnia*. ed. Hugo Kühlewein, vol. 1. Leipzig: 1894.
__, *Hippocrates*. CMG I 1 . ed. J. Heiberg. Leipzig and Berlin: 1927.
__, *Hippocratis de carnibus*. ed. Karl Deichgräber. Leipzig and Berlin: 1935.
__, *Die Hippokratische Schrift Prognostikon*. ed. B. Alexanderson. Göteborg: 1963.
__ ,Hippocrates*Über Achtmonatskinder, Über das Siebenmonatskind (unecht)*. ed. Hermann Grensemann. CMG I 2,1. Berlin: 1968.
__, *Hippocratis De aere aquis locis*. ed. Hans Diller. CMG I 1,2. Berlin: 1970.
__, *Hippocratis De Superfetatione*. ed. Cay Lienau. CMG I 2,2. Berlin 1973.
__, *Hippocratis De natura hominis*. ed. Jacques Jouanna. CMG I 1,3. Berlin: 1975.
__, *Ippocrate, Epidemie Libro Sesto*. a cura di Daniela Manetti e Amneris Roselli. Florence: 1982 (*Biblioteca di Studi Superiori* LXVI).
__, *Hippocrate, Des Vents. De l'Art*. ed. J. Jouanna, Budé V.1. Paris: 1988.
Irigoin, Jacques. "Le rôle des recentiores dans l' etablissement du texte hippocratique," *Corpus Hippocraticum, Colloque de Mons*, ed. R. Joly. Mons 1977.
Jaeger, Werner. *Diokles von Karystos*. Berlin: 1938.
Jouanna, Jacques. "L' Analyse codicologique du Parisinus gr. 2140 et l' histoire du texte hippocratique." *Scriptorium* 38 (1984) 50-67.
Kahn, Charles. "Democritus and the Origins of Moral Psychology." *AJP* 106 (1985) 1-31.
Karl Kalbfleisch. "Medizinische Texte." *Berliner Klassikertexte* III (1905) 5-9.

Kind, Friedrich Ernst. "Krateuas." RE XI 2 (1922) 1644-5.
Koenen, Ludwig, and Reinhold Merkelbach, "Apollodoros (περὶ θεῶν), Epicharm und die Meropis," in Hanson, A., *Collectanea Papyrologica I*, pp. 1-26.
Kollesch, Jutta Harig-. "Zeuxis" *Die kleine Pauly* Vol. 5 (Munich: 1975) 1527.
Kudlien, Fridolf. "Paetus." RE Suppl. 10 (1965) 473-4.
__, "Zeuxis." RE II 19 (1972) 386-7.
__, "Medical Ethics and Popular Ethics," *Clio Medica* 5 (1970) 107-111.
Kühlewein, H. *Hippocratis opera quae feruntur omnia*. Vol. 1, Leipzig: 1894. Prolegomena by Johannes Ilberg.
Lasserre, François and Ph. Mudry (edd). *Formes de pensée dans la collection hippocratique. Actes du IVe colloque international hippocratique* (Lausanne 21-26 septembre 1981). Geneva: 1983.
Lewin, Arnold H. *Hippocrates Visits Democritus: Letters 10-17 of the Hippocratic Corpus*. Tr. with intro. and notes. M.A. Diss. Cornell: 1968.
Lonie, Iain. *The Hippocratic Treatises 'On Generation', 'On the Nature of the Child', 'Diseases IV.'* Ars Medica II.7. Berlin: 1981.
Marcks, Johann F. *Symbola critica ad epistolographos Graecos*. Diss. Bonn: 1883.
Martin, Victor. "Une recueil de diatribes cyniques: Pap. Gen. 271," *Museum Helveticum* 16 (1969) 77-117.
Michelini, Ann. " 'ΥΒΡΙΣ and Plants," *HSCP* 82 (1978) 35-44.
Momigliano, Arnaldo. "Una lettera a Claudio e una lettera ad Antigona Gonata". *Athenaeum* 11 (1933) 132-135.
Mondolfo, R. and L. Taran, *Eraclito, Testimonianze e Imitazioni*. Florence: 1972.
Morel, R. "Pharmakopoles." RE XIX 2 (1939) 1840-1.
Nachmanson, Ernst. *Erotiani Vocum Hippocraticum collectio*. Uppsala: 1918.
__, *Erotianstudien*. Uppsala: 1917.
Paton, W. R., and Hicks, E. L. *The Inscriptions of Cos*. Oxford: 1891.
Peek, Werner. *Griechische Vers-inschriften I*. Berlin: 1955.
Petersen, Christian. "Zeit und Lebensverhältnisse des Hippokrates." *Philologus* 4 (1849) 209-265.
Philippson, Robert. "Verfasser und Abfassungzeit der sogenannte Hippokrates-briefe." *Rheinisches Museum* 77 (1928) 293-328.
Pickard-Cambridge, Arthur W. *The Dramatic Festivals of Athens*. Oxford: 1953.
Pigeaud, Jackie, *La maladie de l'âme*. Paris: 1981.
Pinault, Jody Rubin, *Biographical Fiction in the Lives of Hippocrates*. Diss., University of Penna. 1983.
__, "How Hippocrates cured the Plague," *J. Hist. Med. and Allied Sciences* 41 (1986) 52-75.
Pohlenz, Max. "Zu den hippokratischen Briefen," *Hermes* 52 (1917) 348-353.
Pomtow, Heinrich. "Delphische Neufunde III. Hippokrates und die Asklepiaden in Delphi." *Klio* 15 (1918) 303-338.
Robert, Louis. "Décret des Asclépiastes de Kolophon." *Revue des Études Ancienne* 28 (1926) 7-9.
__, "Décret des Asclépiastes de Kolophon." *Revue de Philologie* Ser. 3., 8 (1934) 272-4.

Sabatucci, A. "Alcune note sulle epistole di Chione," *Studi Italiani di filologia classica* 14 (1906) 374-414.

Sakalis, Dimitrios Th. "Beiträge zu den pseudo-hippokratischen Briefen." in *Formes de pensée dans la collection hippocratique*, ed. F. Lasserre and P. Mudry. (Geneva:1983) pp. 499-514.

Scarborough, John, and Vivian Nutton. "The Preface of Dioscorides' *Materia Medica*: Introduction, Translation, Commentary," *Transactions and Studies of the College of Physicians of Philadelphia* 4 (1982) 187-227.

Schneider, K. E. C. "Hippokrates und Artaxerxes." *Janus* 1 (1846) 86-115.

Segre, Mario. "Grano di Tessaglia a Coo." *Rivista di Filologia e d' Istruzione Classica* N.S. 12 (1934) 169-193.

Sherwin-White, Susan M. *Ancient Cos.* Göttingen: 1978.

Smith, Wesley D. *The Hippocratic Tradition.* Ithaca and London: 1979.

__, "Notes on Ancient Medical Historiography." *BHM* 63 (1989) 73-109.

Sokolowski, Franciszek. *Lois sacrées des cités grecques*, Supplement. Paris: 1962.

Stuart, Zeph. "Democritus and the Cynics." *Harvard Studies in Classical Philology* 63 (1958) 179-191.

Sykutris, J. "Epistolographie." RE Suppl. 5 (1931) 185-220.

Temkin, Owsei, "Hippocrates as the Physician of Democritus," *Gesnerus* 42 (1985) 455-464.

Wellmann, Max. *Krateuas. Abh. könig. Gesellschaft zu Göttingen*, Phil-hist. Kl., N. F. 3, Nr. 1. Berlin: 1897.

__, *Die Fragmente der sikilischen Aerzte Akron, Philistion, und des Diokles von Karystos.* Berlin: 1901.

__, *Pedanii Dioscoridis Anazarbei De materia medica.* Berlin: 1907-14.

__, *Hippokratesglossare. Quellen und Studien zur Geschichte der Naturwissenschaften und der Medizin* 2. Berlin:1931.

Wilson, Nigel G. *Scholars of Byzantium.* Oxford: 1983.

INDEX